ADVANCE PRAISE FOR

Pregnant Pause

"*Pregnant Pause* is insightful, touching and incredibly funny. Carrie Friedman finally gives a voice to the non-pregnant and persecuted! If you're looking for refuge from the pressure of prying questions, pet substitution and the call of your biologic clock, her sharp wit is a hilarious diversion."

—Adrianne Frost, author of
I Hate Other People's Kids

"A very honest, personal, and humorous exploration of one woman's pre-pregnancy journey."

—Christie Mellor, author of
The Three-Martini Playdate

"Carrie Friedman is an absolute delight!"

—Jamie Cat Callan, author of
*French Women Don't Sleep Alone:
Pleasurable Secrets to Finding Love*

Pregnant Pause

My Journey Through Obnoxious Questions,
Baby Lust, Meddling Relatives, and
Pre-Partum Depression

Carrie Friedman

CITADEL PRESS
Kensington Publishing Corp.
www.kensingtonbooks.com

CITADEL PRESS BOOKS are published by

Kensington Publishing Corp.
850 Third Avenue
New York, NY 10022

All Kensington titles, imprints, and distributed lines are available at special
quantity discounts for bulk purchases for sales promotions, premiums, fund-
raising, educational, or institutional use. Special book excerpts or customized
printings can also be created to fit specific needs. For details, write or phone
the office of the Kensington special sales manager: Kensington Publishing
Corp., 850 Third Avenue, New York, NY 10022, attn: Special Sales Department;
phone 1-800-221-2647.

Names and identifying characteristics have been changed to protect people's
privacy without damaging the integrity of the narrative.

First printing: April 2009

10 9 8 7 6 5 4 3 2 1

Printed in the United States of America

Library of Congress Control Number 2008942168

ISBN-13: 978-0-8065-3116-8
ISBM-10: 0-8065-3116-9

For my parents

Contents

Pregnant Pause

The Dreaded Question

"So . . . ? When are the babies coming?"

I had been married all of five minutes, and this was the only thing my third cousin twice removed, whom I'd never met but my mother insisted we invite, had to say to me: not "beautiful ceremony," not "I hope you and your brand new husband are happy forever," not "Hey, I'm your third cousin twice removed. Nice to meet you."

"I thought I'd eat my cake first," I said, and laughed it off.

But as the night progressed, three more people asked *me*—not my husband, mind you—when we were going to hop on the baby train.

I spent three hundred days planning a disposable evening that was mostly for our guests; I got carpal tunnel syndrome handwriting everyone's place card in calligraphy, seated enemies far away from each other, ordered flowers and cake that no one's allergic to, booked music the guests would like, and bought party favors, even though I felt the $220 dinner per guest was party favor enough. And they were asking me about babies?

1

Couldn't I enjoy a couple of hours celebrating the latest milestone in my life without being prodded about the next? And why was everyone asking about babies? Why was no one asking about my career, which was far more important to me at that point in my life?

At the time, it was only mildly irritating. They were probably just trying to make conversation. It was my wedding night! I was in my twenties! We had time!

Since our wedding three years ago, with every anniversary we've celebrated, people have asked more questions. And each time they've asked, I've fallen deeper into what I'm calling my pre-partum depression.

I've always planned to have kids and still do. But as it's inching closer to becoming a reality, I've become paralyzed by fear, which makes a lot of sense, considering it's one of the biggest decisions a person can make. (But no pressure, right?) For as much as I love children, I worry they might ruin life as I've known it.

I couldn't find anyone else who could relate, as most of my friends were at different stages—already parents or still

---

Pre-Partum Depression: Noun

A state of fear, anxiety, uncertainty, and/or hopelessness about the prospect of becoming (or deciding to become) a parent; sometimes manifested physiologically by increased heart rate, sweating, hives induced by ill-behaved children and their worse-behaved parents, and stalling, causing the sufferer sleeplessness, irritability, dry mouth, and greater potential to be unapproachable at parties and other social functions.

See also: irreversible decision.

single. I searched for books on the topic but didn't find any that supported or quelled my feelings.

In all the women's magazines and websites, no category exists for what I'm going through. "Planning for Baby," in women's media, means articles about what to register for, how many onesies you'll really need, and all the ways to predict when you're ovulating. No mention of the self-doubt and the fears of how drastically it'll alter *everything*—career, marriage, finances. There are sections for health, diet and fitness, pregnancy, infertility, beauty, and style. Where's the section called "Thinking About Having a Baby?" or "Just Married—Now What?" There isn't even a "marriage" section; there's "weddings," which shouldn't surprise us much, since a lot of people focus on the wedding and not enough on the actual marriage. (Hence, a 50 percent divorce rate, perhaps?) Planning for a baby isn't about stuff, as most of us know. It's not about the shower or the pretty pastel nursery. It's about the most important and challenging job anyone can ever choose to take on: raising a healthy, balanced child in today's turbulent world and deciding whether you're ready to accept the challenge.

With so little to guide me in my struggle, I assumed I was alone on this. Boy was I wrong.

In 2007, I wrote a personal essay published in *Newsweek* called "Stop Setting Alarms on My Biological Clock," addressing my anxiety about starting a family and the near constant badgering to join the parent "hood." Almost immediately, e-mails poured in. The majority were overwhelmingly positive from like-minded individuals who had similar concerns and misgivings about parenthood. Some felt bullied into having kids by family, friends, or society. Others, who had trouble conceiving, explained the devastation they were forced to relive every time someone asked them when they were finally going to have kids. I heard from couples who were waiting as long as possible and from some who didn't want kids at all. I spoke with many parents who were outraged by their sometimes fanatic hyper-parenting counterparts (and I heard from a few of those fanatic hyper-parenting counterparts as well, some of whom e-mailed to wish me infertility, divorce, and—I'm not kidding—death in childbirth). I was shocked by how many people had stories to tell. So many people were terrified, just like I was, of taking that next huge step. So many of them felt secretly ashamed or suffered in silence because, after all, people had babies every day.

Was there something wrong with us—a group of people who didn't want to have babies, couldn't have babies, or had different priorities from the mainstream when it came to raising a family? Why was no one addressing our concerns or us?

Over the last few years, I've been chronicling my struggles with this issue. *Pregnant Pause* is for anyone who has or has had some reservations about parenthood and its culture and is reaching out for solidarity. We'll explore some contributing factors to pre-partum depression (in the order I personally experienced them): from annoyance (stop asking me that dreaded question!) to baby lust (my last childless friend just told me she's pregnant!) to disenchantment (can a person truly have it all? And seriously, don't kids learn manners anymore?) to everything in between. You'll hear from the people I interviewed from all walks of life: women, men, couples, single people, married people, partners, teachers, gynecologists, psychiatrists, people who have kids, people who want to have kids, and people who don't want to have kids.

This book is in no way meant to be an attack on parents.

Parenting is a tough job, no doubt. It's recognition of this that contributes to some of my fear. Rather, this book is an examination of all the aspects of parenthood that can (and should) give a person pause and provides a voice for a group of us who haven't been heard from yet. I hope you'll find support and comfort in the pages ahead.

CHAPTER ONE

The Baby Train

> *Making the decision to have a child is momentous. It is to decide forever to have your heart go walking around outside your body.*
> —ELIZABETH STONE

It was our third hour at the Uffizi Gallery in Florence, Italy, and my husband, Stephen, was practically making love to his audio guide, a long telephonic device he held to his ear and listened to as if the female recording was whispering sweet nothings to him. If he could French-kiss her he would have.

We were in a fight. Over breakfast at our hotel that morning, Stephen read in an American newspaper that men also had a biological clock. He then went on to say, quite casually, that he'd like us to "hop on the baby train sooner rather than later."

For him to say this aloud meant he'd been thinking about it a great deal. Stephen's a brilliant writer; he does

not throw words around. The newspaper article was probably just the cherry on the sundae.

"WHAT?" I shrieked so loud you'd think I just found a
roach in my Flakes di Frosted.

The explanation for my scream was simple: we had said
we would wait. For the last two years, we'd been enjoying
each other, traveling as much as possible and focusing on
our careers. Twelve years Stephen's junior, I had assumed
my youth was a gift: we could put off having kids longer
than most of his friends, who by now were in their forties
and saddled with three or four children.

Not once did I consider how it must be for Stephen to
have no child-free friends left—no one to go out to movies
with at the last minute or out for drinks and a guy chat because most of them coached their kids' little league games
after work or raced home to spell the wife while she took a
much-needed rest. I never thought about how this was af-
fecting him.

"Am I holding you back?" I asked him, as we took an
after-breakfast stroll through the Piazza del Duomo.

Stephen thought about this. (He had to think about it!)

"No," he said, a little too hesitantly for my taste. "But if
we start now, I'll only be 59 when the kid graduates from
high school."

My heart sank. Another side of his struggle I hadn't even
thought about—his age and issues with mortality. I'm an
awful wife, but, in my defense, it's easy to forget Stephen's
age because he's so young at heart, runs ten miles a day,
and takes care of himself so well.

I'm reminded of this fact as we climbed Giotto's bell
tower—all 280 feet of it. I tried to keep up with him as he
took the steps two at a time. Meanwhile, I lost feeling in

both my arms. Between my huffing and puffing, I told him, "This isn't a unilateral decision, you know."

"Oh, I know," he said. "Hence, we don't have kids yet."

Had he been making concessions all this time? And if so, why didn't he speak up sooner?

"But I'm not yet 30!" I said, pausing on the seemingly never-ending stairway to a view of Florence that had better the hell be worth it. "I've got a lot of life left to lead!"

"It's not a degenerative illness, Carrie. It's having a kid."

He had a point. Why did I associate having children with an end point? I've always loved kids, yet I felt like I'd be giving up my own life in order to bring another one into the world.

"I think I'm going to throw up," I said, and sat on the steps in the dark, mildewy stairwell. I felt a swirling, all-encompassing nausea. If my fingers and toes could throw up, they would have. Believe me, it wasn't the heat or the stairs. It was terror. Suddenly, I was seeing stars. And plastic primary-colored baby equipment littering our custom-designed living room back home. I saw spit-up in my hair and on my shirts. I saw my computer and social life collecting dust.

As we photographed the bronze doors of the Baptistery, I thought about how different it was for men. They could say casually, over eggs in a foreign country, that it was time to bite the bullet and start a family, and that was it. For a woman, it was to say good-bye to her life and body and career as she once knew it. Everything will be turned upside down. And while I've always wanted to have children, would I ever fully be ready to give my life over to that kind of insanity? Stephen could go back to work the day after the birth if he wanted. He could escape.

Right before we left for our Italian adventure, Stephen got a phone call from one of his best friends who told him he and his wife had their baby that morning. My husband asked the name, weight, and details. Not two seconds after the baby information was imparted, the friend changed the topic and started discussing Battlestar Galactica and the latest exciting episode. I couldn't believe it! For a second, I thought it was a different phone call with someone else. But it was the same friend. They talked for twenty minutes about Battlestar Galactica. Now look, I know it's a great show, but the man just became a father. Was the TV show really that good?

When my husband got off the phone, I asked who brought it up. He said his friend did. I was shocked. His wife, I guaranteed, hadn't had a conversation of that nature—a normal conversation—since giving birth and probably wouldn't for the next four months. All her conversations would be about breastfeeding, sleeping, pumping and will include lovely words like nipples and engorged. If a female friend of mine told me she'd had a child earlier that day and I basically said in response, "Cool! Hey, did you catch Grey's Anatomy last night?" I'd be unfriended swiftly and for good reason.

Someone told me that men almost need to talk about something else in order to convince themselves and others that nothing has changed. Yet the mothers are forced to face this change head-on, with baby and breast pumps suddenly replacing all the time they had to watch TV, let alone brush their teeth. Stephen's life will go back to normal in a matter of days—he'll return to the office and go about his routine. But my career will take a brief hiatus at best, and at worst, it'll disintegrate entirely as I learn a new vocabulary of baby words. Stephen can play tennis the same week I deliver, should he so choose, whereas I'll be a waddling mess of leaky fluids.

Looking up at the stunning cupola del Brunelleschi in the cathedral, I whisper-yelled at Stephen, "Well of course you're ready to have kids! You won't be the one who has to take care of them!" Even my whispers echoed off the walls.

"Oh yeah?" Stephen whisper-yelled right back, "And who does all the cooking, Carrie?"

If this were a movie, all the action in the cathedral would grind to a halt to the tune of a scratching record.

True. Stephen does all the cooking. It's not that I'm a terrible cook—you have to do something a fair amount in order to know you're bad at it. It's that I don't cook. Stephen loves to cook so much that he gets flushed when explaining how to clarify butter. More than twice, I've turned TV dinners over onto plates and tried to pass them off as home cooked. I've never fooled him.

"What are we gonna feed the kids, Carrie, Balance Bars?" Stephen asked.

Salt on the wound. Balance Bars have been my breakfast food of choice for the last five years and, let's face it, dinner food when he was working late.

"No!" I said defensively, all the while secretly wondering, what's so wrong with Balance Bars? It's balanced nutrition! I can think of worse foods kids could eat.

For a while, I thought I was allergic to the physical act of cooking because I was so repulsed by the idea of it. It's been a joke at family dinners of how infrequently I cook, and Christmas gifts often include aprons, cookbooks, and pie dishes as "subtle" hints.

I promise you, it's not just laziness. I don't want to know how to cook. Why? Am I afraid it'll instantly turn me into June Cleaver? No, of course not. Am I afraid it will automat-

ically fall on me every night? No, not really. Am I afraid I'll
turn into my mother? Bingo. Having watched my mother
cook and clean for all of us for decades, I vowed not to
learn. Of course, I threw the baby out with the bathwater
and now wish I had some basic skills. I only know how to
make macaroni and macaroni-related casseroles: Mac 'n
Peas, Mac 'n Corn, Mac 'n Tuna, and Cheezy Mac, my signature dish and a Carrie Friedman adaptation of Hamburger
Helper's Cheeseburger Macaroni.

My father would come home from work and, like most fa-
thers at the time, would play with the kids, read the paper,
enjoy his TV programs, and eat my mother's dinner.

As kids, we observed this. I remember thinking that if I
had to choose between roles, I'd want my father's because
I wanted to do whatever I wished after dinner too, like
playing outside or watching Punky Brewster. My mother
never made us help with the dishes, and in retrospect, I
wish she had. But she was doing what she thought she was
supposed to do—her wifely and motherly duties. My sister,
I would later find out, took away a similar lesson. We're
really good at waiting to be served or setting the table, but
as far as cooking's concerned, we're mostly clueless. (And
we're not doing a whole lot to pursue it now either.)

We would later figure out that we feared we, too, would
be relegated to the kitchen. We knew our mother was a
brilliant woman with advanced degrees and a full-time
job. There she was, cleaning up after her family. I would
later, in college, identify my discomfort when I learned
about the gender ideologies that placed these tasks on
women's backs. These gender roles were added on top of a
full day's work. This was the 1980s and early '90s, long after
The Feminine Mystique came out. Did motherhood ensure
that this would happen? Would I become one of those

mothers with a dazed look in her eyes that came from exhaustion, unfulfilled dreams, the "problem that had no
name" described by Betty Friedan, or all of the above?

Standing in the Uffizi gallery again, Stephen and I were
in a standoff. He listened to his audio chick and I sat on a
bench, writing notes and hyperventilating. It must have
been "unruly kids" day at the museum, as they were everywhere I looked.

The kids screamed at their parents, hit their mothers,
and arched their backs as they threw tantrums on the
floor, all done beneath priceless works of art. The parents
looked worn out, especially the moms, who had dark circles under their eyes and gray skin and wrinkles from
frowning so much. I was tired just looking at them.

Stephen stopped listening to his audio whore when he
spotted me sitting on the bench. He came over and told
me, "You embody the joke about the American who pulls
up to the Louvre and says, 'Which way to the Mona Lisa?
I'm double parked.'"

I wasn't proud of this, but I was also no longer ashamed
of the fact that I didn't love museums. I've always found
them overwhelming. There's no way I could possibly take
in all that art.

I pointed out the miserable parents and their horrible
kids. "You're projecting," Stephen said. "They don't look
that unhappy to me, Carrie." We see what we want to see.

Stephen and I had been married for a little over two
years, after dating for less than a year. Now we were so far
past the "come here oftens" of dating that it felt like another life ago, in a way that made me both relieved and
nostalgic. In that other life, we had agreed that we'd wait
to have kids in order to enjoy each other, our careers, and
our travels. Now it felt like he had turned on me.

"What about our three-year plan?" I asked him. "Remember, we were going to travel and have as much fun as possible before we started a family?"

He gestured to the museum behind us. "We go on a couple trips a year and we're almost at the three-year mark!"

"What are you talking about? Are you counting the time we've been dating too?"

He nodded.

"You can't do that!" I said. "You have to go by how long we've been married!"

I wanted so badly to just come out and tell him I needed more time. I wasn't ready. But I didn't want to dissuade his desire, as I married him partly because I loved the fact he wanted children and was so good with them.

I wandered into the Botticelli room and stared at The Birth of Venus, the goddess with her strawberry blonde tendrils wrapping around her body and covering her nether regions. The story was that Venus emerged from the sea, born a full-grown woman. If only babies were born full-grown and could feed themselves, instead of needing their mother's milk every two hours—no seventh-grade awkwardness to help them through, no threatening to kill their prom dates for standing them up. No. Instead, you got this beautiful (albeit naked) young woman who could help her parents in their advanced age.

As I was navigating through the crowds in the museum, I saw a pack of four moms pushing strollers, looking bone tired and charging toward me like a sleep-deprived version of the four horsemen of the apocalypse.

I turned away, only to be greeted by a painting of a mother holding a baby to her fleshy breast that drooped in the shape of a teardrop. I turned again and looked right at one of Titian's zaftig women lounging on a chaise, her childbearing hips on full display. Everywhere I turned, I felt trapped—Raphael's Madonna del Cardellino: Mary and a baby Christ and a baby John the Baptist, but from where I was standing, at first, it looked like twins. Good lord, there was a truly horrific thought.

I sneaked into another room. Caravaggio. Surely, Caravaggio could calm me down. But instead, I stared at his oil on canvas mounted on wood depiction of Medusa. The snakes were tangled and Medusa's eyes were wild and a little bloodshot. Crazy eyes. Now granted, she had snakes for hair—I'd be a little out of sorts myself. This is what I'll surely turn into, stretched too thin as my toddler thinks it's funny to poop on the carpet. I'll be reduced to shuttling kids to the mall and buying them cell phones when they're six.

I looked away and found that the stroller apocalypse was back on my tail. I hid behind a pillar out of their way and tried to catch my breath, only to realize I was in front of Michelangelo's David. Heavenly. I overheard two women checking him out:

"I'd like a piece of that ass."

"He's so fine he's *foyne*."

I smiled and nodded.

My hoodie stuck to my back with sweat in the unair-conditioned gallery. I forgot to convert the Italian temperature into Fahrenheit, so my corduroy pants and sweatshirt were melting me in the ninety-degree heat. I was beginning to smell like a Sbarro's restaurant.

After I left my post behind the pillar, I spotted Stephen looking at a painting of the Annunciation and nodding. What was he nodding about? Did he "get" it? What was to get? Did my judgments make me ignorant or did my igno-

rance make me judgmental? I looked at it myself: the angel
Gabriel knelt before Mary, telling her she would conceive a
child to be born the son of God. In this version, her facial
expression was different from all the other paintings of the
Annunciation I had seen. In this one, her head was slightly
cocked, her eyes the slightest bit squinty in disbelief, as if
to say, "Whatchu talkin' about, Willis?" Of course, I was
probably projecting.

I couldn't stop thinking about how much my life would
change once we had a family. I'd be pulling all-nighters,
my body mushy and dimply. I'd live my life in sweatpants,
cleaning up various fluids. It was mostly mother's work.
Dads came home at night, swooped the child into the air
with their fresh arms and became the hero. That was how
it was when I was a kid: mom was the bad cop because she
was with us more. She did most of the heavy lifting—the
mundane household chores, helping us with homework,
and the difficult task of disciplining three children who
were very close in age. Dad was at work, which was in no
way easy either, and though my mother worked too, I always felt as if she envied him for getting to spend more
time out of the house, as her work hours were abbreviated
because she had to take care of the kids.

A couple wandering around in the Botticelli room held
hands as they whispered to each other. Probably a third
date. *They will get married,* I decided. And in less than five
years, they could become Stephen and me: at separate
ends of the museum, enjoying things at very different
paces. I was officially an "after" picture.

I searched for Stephen, and when I found him across the
room, for a split second, I didn't recognize him. Who was
this man? This was the man I was spending the rest of my
life with? Raising kids with? Did he wonder the same thing

about me? *Who is this woman I married? And why has she been going through a Unabomber fashion phase?* (I'd been wearing a lot of hooded sweatshirts.) We'd reached the point in our marriage where I was annoyed by the way he slurped his soup, and he had figured out that when I didn't wear eye makeup I looked like a fetus. All bets were off.

On this trip, I had only been aware of our differences. I cried during the emotional denouements of any and every movie, even if it was *Big Momma's House*. He rarely cried about anything, which made me wonder if he was detached. He didn't like sports, whereas I structured my weekends around them. He ran away from arguments when I wanted to crack them wide open. At times, no one in the world could irritate me as much: I hated when he Saran wrapped a single bite of food and called it "leftovers," when he referred to a family as a "gang," when he mashed his face into a bag of movie popcorn like it was a trough.

These were, of course, small things, and I was neglecting to mention the things we had in common, which, fortunately, weren't small. But love and life were in the details, right? Will we prove too different to sustain our marriage? Should we be with people who go through museums at the same pace? Maybe he was better off with the natural beauty over there wearing sandals with socks. She was probably someone who not only knew how to cook but did so with the freshest organic ingredients.

But then I remembered how I dated plenty of sports fans or emotional poet types, and invariably there were other things missing. Big things, like chemistry, sense of humor, and fidelity. Sure, they shared my love of dogs dressed up as humans, but they also owned guns or voted for Bush.

After a bit of thinking, I joined Stephen beside yet another portrait of a woman who had been dead since the sixteenth century. He wrapped his arms around me and pointed at a little boy—the only well-behaved kid in the whole place—and whispered, "We could do that!" And the way he said it, with so much joy and certainty, reminded me of why I loved him, his hazel eyes with starbursts in the middle, so excited and full of hope. For a moment, the idea of doing anything, including raising a child, with this man by my side, sounded like the best idea I'd ever heard.

But as much as I loved how primed my husband was to have children, I had to be primed too. I knew girlfriends who had kids before they were completely ready, and I could say with as much certainty that there was nothing worse than an ambivalent or emotionally unprepared mother.

"Can we start trying when I'm 30? Can you wait just another year?"

"It's a deal," he said.

"I'm just sort of pissed off," I said to my therapist upon returning from our Italian adventure.

"Why?" he asked, his pen poised to take notes.

"I'm pissed at the fact that my body, my life, all of it will be turned over to this child. Will it consume me?"

"Yes," my therapist said.

"Wow. Way to sugarcoat it," I said. "Thanks."

I knew motherhood would begin another chapter—hell, a whole new book—of my life. But I really liked the book I was reading at the time. Still, I saw it as an ending, instead of a glorious beginning. Having kids is about sacrifice. And I'm not talking about the obvious sacrifices—of sleep, of routine, of freedom. These all come with the lengthy job description listed under "parent."

My therapist told me I'd know when I was ready to start a family. He said I would feel it in my bones.

I wanted to ask for my money back. I could have gotten cheaper, less ambiguous advice from a Magic 8-ball.

His advice reminded me of my least favorite saying, "What's meant to be is meant to be," or its slightly less lame but still wishy-washy cousin: "Everything happens for a reason."

"Part of preparing for parenthood is letting go," he told me. "Surrendering control."

"Yikes!" I said. I'd been white-knuckling most aspects of my life for as long as I could remember.

And my therapist knew me well enough to nod and say, "Yeah. I know." His brow furrowed, and he shrugged a little, as if to add, "You are so screwed, sister."

CHAPTER TWO

Bump Watch

*You should never say anything to a woman
that even remotely suggests that you think
she's pregnant unless you can see an actual
baby emerging from her at that moment.*
—DAVE BARRY

During my first three years of marriage, everywhere I went, people's eyes migrated to my unchanging waistline. And it was everyone, not just friends and family, but the eye doctor, the dental assistant, the bagger at the grocery store. All of them felt entitled to ask.

The strangest inquiry had to have been from my yoga teacher. I drove across town once a week to take this class because I loved the teacher, a hip young German woman with a thick accent who'd play Tina Turner music during the sun salutations. She was the kind of funky that made you wish you had a tattoo: something small and tasteful but a little bit bad. Because she hadn't fully grasped the language yet, she was often unintentionally poetic when

21

speaking to all of us. My favorite was, "You are lifting the springtime of your heart to the flowers in your skull."

I was resting in savasana pose, on my back, when she knelt down near my ear and said in a whisper, "Your ovaries are ripe, yes?"

I opened my eyes and looked up at her. "My what?" Surely she meant something else. Eggs? Omelettes? Oranges? Or maybe this was some sort of German lesbian come-on line?

She whispered again, "Your ovaries, they are bright and ready for the babies."

I pulled my legs to my chest, as if this could somehow block her X-ray vision into my pelvis, and stared at her, confused. Who was this woman, and why was she tracking my ovulation better than I was? How could she tell? Was I bloated? And did she have to interrupt my peaceful resting pose, the one chance I had per week to fully relax and reflect?

I didn't stick around after class to clarify, and my ovaries and I never went back.

The Tent Dress

Multiple Choice:
You do extra abdominal work at the gym because:

a. It's good for you.
b. You saw the latest Madonna video and are jealous of her abnormally rock-hard abs.
c. You want to lessen the chances that someone will mistake the slightest tummy bump as a baby bump.

If you answered *c*, then you're probably as mad as I am about this baby-doll dress craze. I have actually shed tears in Bloomingdales, searching for anything with a normal waist, reasoning that I do not work so hard on my abdominals (ab-fab class twice a week so that the next day it hurts to laugh or breathe) to wear a dress that's essentially a poncho. No wonder people constantly asked when the baby was due. Because everyone looks pregnant in a high-waisted garment.

How did this happen? When did Shakespearean fashion come back into style? I've seen myself in empire-waisted dresses, and at best, I look like Lady Macbeth. If you throw a beret and kneesocks on me, I'd be the bard himself. Who thought this would be attractive, and who can tell me where to send my angry letter? When the fashion industry declared the return of the muumuu during Fall Fashion Week a few years ago, they tried to make it hip and trendy. Yeah, it's hip and trendy if you're a six-foot-tall-anorexic supermodel. But for the rest of us, the muumuu is just a muumuu.

These dresses always make me look wider than I am tall, expansive, like a tent with campers in it. (Note to designers everywhere: anything that's called a "bubble dress" is just a bad idea.) Because of this fad, my tailor and I've had a very close relationship. Every other week, I'm bringing him a baby doll dress or a loose-fitting blouse to take *way* in.

But even when you finally find a form-fitting outfit, you're still going to have to deal with people who think it's their business to poke and prod you about your plans to procreate.

On our first Thanksgiving as a married couple, a mere

month after Stephen and I tied the knot, my Great-Uncle Marvin focused on the area just below my waistline and said, "Oh Carrie! I see a little paunch! Is somebody expecting?" His eyes became googly, and he sounded like he was talking to a puppy. He didn't go so far as to poke my paunch, which was fortunate since I'd have broken his fingers.

"No, Marv," I said. "I just finished eating Thanksgiving dinner, just like you." I stopped short of asking him when *he* was due.

Why did people feel entitled to ask? Did they see the wedding band and connect marriage with babies? It was obnoxious—for all he knew, I couldn't have kids. For all *I* knew I couldn't have kids, as I hadn't yet tried. But imagine if I had submitted to all kinds of treatments, only to come up empty-wombed. Imagine how painful this line of interrogation would be. Stephen thinks some people ask because it helps them validate their own choices. But he doesn't truly understand how infuriating it is, and that's no doubt because nobody badgers men about procreativity with the same frequency.

Was there a more personal question than the equivalent to, "So! You and the hubby having lots of unprotected sex lately?" How would they feel if I looked at their wrinkles and gray hair and said, "You look older every time I see you. You planning for your funeral yet?" or "You're menopausal, right? How's the dryness?" Sure, maybe they were just making conversation, but when I thought of icebreakers, birth control didn't spring to mind.

Perhaps child-free couples should all carry a printed card in their wallets, with this list of possible responses to the dreaded "when are you having babies?" question:

"My wife and I have been married for 6 years now, and for the first 4 years, everyone, even total strangers, have interrogated my wife on why we haven't had kids yet. Then when they find out we've had problems getting pregnant, they offer unsolicited advice on how to increase our chances of pregnancy even as far as suggesting a surrogate. It's like there is a rule stating that immediately after getting married, you have a time deadline to have a baby or you may be penalized. The awareness that you may not be able to bear children is already stressful, but having everyone else expecting you to have children ASAP is so overwhelming, we just want to punch someone and tell them to shut up. The pressure is usually on her because she's the baby machine, so therefore she's the one at fault. I feel so terrible for her. She gets the brunt of all the flack. I truly wish the world wouldn't put so many expectations on women to have children as a standard to compare everyone else to. Society can be cruel though they think they're being helpful."

—P.R., Fresno, CA

- "I had two this morning. They were delicious."
- "Actually, I can't have kids. I'd managed to go a few hours without thinking about it, but thanks for reminding me."
- "Well, we had one. You must not have read about it, but long story short, don't hire an English nanny."
- "We're not. We've decided to clone."

Depending on the circumstances, you may have to adjust your responses to fit the asker of such questions. While a high level of sarcasm is appropriate for skeevy great-uncles and prying colleagues, it isn't necessarily appropriate for your mother.

Odds are, your mom means well and you love her to death, but you want to find a kind way to say, "Get a hobby besides tuning into womb-watch 2009!"

For years, my mother has called me with news of her latest purchases for "The Baby Drawer." The first time this happened I was a freshman in college. My sister was a senior. Babies weren't even on the horizon. Still, my mother would explain how she was buying a gift for someone and came across "the most precious little cardigan with strawberries sewn on and matching bloomers and strawberry buttons. Strawberry buttons, Carrie! I had to get it for the drawer. And you know they had the same thing with sailboats for a boy, of course."

She said she bought these items "just in case." Just in case what? I once asked her. You mean if one of her unattached daughters got knocked up accidentally? Did she think the end of the world was coming? Was there a baby clothes shortage?

"You never know," she said, "if these adorable pieces will be around in a hundred years when you and your sister finally decide to have kids."

Since then, that drawer in my parents' home has spilled into an entire dresser. And when my sister and I both got married, the baby stuff outgrew the dresser and took over a whole closet.

Whenever my sister and I are home for major holidays, we poke around in the baby closet. The shelves are full of white cardboard boxes that look like bakery boxes. Inside are different kinds of sweets: delicate soft blues and pinks and warm yellows. These are not just pieces of clothing. No. They are whole sets—hats that match sweaters that

"Maybe I'll encourage my mother to adopt her own new kids the next time she complains about having no grandkids. Maybe I'll encourage my sister to shop for her dogs rather than comment on all the things she'll buy if I ever have kids. Maybe I'll just laugh and say, 'Why should I have kids? After all, yours are annoying enough for the whole planet.'"

—B.K., Lawrence, KS

match little corduroy pants. Shoes for girls in a row, shoes for boys in a row, a baby-sized pimp coat, snowsuits for every age, and a baby fedora. As much as we know this is mom's way of enticing us to get pregnant already, we still sometimes fall prey to it.

"I am so calling dibs on the strawberry sweater set," my sister says to me. "And the fedora. Just an FYI."

"I will fight you for both," I say. "It's on, bitch."

At some point, my mom stopped mentioning each purchase for the baby closet. She picked up on our cues that questions about procreation weren't welcome. Subtle hints, like "Stop asking me when I'm going to have a baby" and "We will have kids when we're good and ready, thanks."

If you have a similar situation with your mother and your responses are still falling on deaf ears, then consider some of the other tried and true diffusing techniques I've learned after years and years of inadvertent research (see the box on the next page).

In addition to the baby closet, my mother has another hobby to keep her busy: she believes the world is out to get every last one of us.

Recent voice mails from my mother include:

"A man died in Los Angeles today and all he was doing

Pre-Partum Pointer: Distract and Redirect

Think of the craziest relative you have and ask about him or her, such as:

- "Mom, does Aunt Minnie still live in her car?"
- "Mom, is Cousin Clark still practicing witchcraft?"
- For a fun variation, try comparing yourself to said crazy relative. "Mom, at least I'm not like Cousin Clark . . ."

If this doesn't spark discussion, then highlight your own cult-related plans:

- "Mom, [insert spouse's name here] and I have decided to join a cult! Isn't that great? You and dad are invited to our next meeting! BYOS—bring your own sacrifice!"

was crossing the street. Make sure you look both ways. And you need to drink more water. It's mom." Click. (As if I might have thought it was someone else.)

"*E. coli* was found in some water in California. Drink bottled only, and you might want to boil it first. It's mom." Click.

My mother is the most Jewish non-Jewish mother in the world. (I'm half-Jewish, so I can say that.) Anxiety is hereditary, and tension is the very life-blood in my family's veins. If we had a family crest, it would be a knight breathing into a paper bag.

Lately, the messages have shifted to news of my former grade school classmates. I'd prefer not to hear about any of them, as they bring back memories of my hopelessly dorky years, when I wore sweater vests. High school ended twelve years ago, and still, some of the names my mother brings up make my skin crawl.

Messages like:

"Well, I ran into Rhona Mandel today at the pedicurist and let me tell you, she has awful feet. Gnarled and just awful. You remember her daughter Jillian, right? The chubby one with the lazy eye, which I guess they got fixed because now she's just *gorgeous* apparently. Anyway. Rhona and her husband are getting"—she lowers her voice to a whisper, as if the Mandels might overhear her in her kitchen—"divorced. But Jillian's pregnant with her third child, Carrie. Her *third*! So, I thought that was nice. Of course, then she asks me about you girls, and I could tell she was wondering if you and your sister can't have kids or something. . . .

Factoid:

In 1975, 1 out of 10 women didn't have children. Today it's 1 out of 5. The census researchers indicate that although they don't directly track the choice factor, they believe the 1 out of 5 today more often reflects the choice not to have children, given that medical technology is so good these days.
    —Laura Carroll, *Families of Two: Interviews with
        Happily Married Couples Without Children by Choice*

Opinionoid: Birthday Parties

Turning one is a big deal, and I will be there with a nice gift for your precious pumpkin, birthday hat firmly fixed on my head. But inviting me to his 2nd, 3rd, and 4th starts to feel a little gift grubby. When will it end? After his bar mitzvah? After her Sweet 16 or 18th? ("Pumpkin can vote now! Hurrah!" Yes, and he can also be emancipated from his parents.)

Anyway, I just wanted to tell you I saw Mrs. Mandel. Honest to God, the ugliest feet you've ever seen in your life.

"Don't eat spinach. It's mom."

Click.

Hands off My Belly

At the birthday party of my friend Reyna's son, Cayden, I made a point of drinking a bottle of beer to avoid any further pregnancy questions. My empire-waisted top (newly tailored and therefore practically a corset) was paired with a skirt so tight I swear you could see the outline of my veins. But Reyna, in full hostess mode, sidled up next to me as her young son, the birthday boy, squirmed out of her embrace. Reyna slipped her cold hand under my shirt. I balked. Before I could push her away, she rubbed my tummy and asked me, concerned: "Why aren't you pregnant yet?"

We were close friends before she had her baby. Ever since then, I wondered why she bothered calling me at all, as she usually spent the entire time on the phone talking to the nanny who was corralling her son, leaving me to end every conversation with some variation of "This is clearly a bad time, I'll let you go," even though she had been the one who called me.

I smiled, broke free from her touch, and headed to the food table to fill said otherwise empty belly with her kid's birthday cake. I didn't know whom to blame: my once good friend who seemed to have lost her manners and tact when she had a baby, or the idiotic bastard who thought the empire waist was due for a comeback.

Cayden, the birthday boy, had registered for his second birthday. Amazing that he knew he just *had* to have that

Mommy & Me fitness DVD and the Burberry plaid overalls, perfect for the holidays. Impeccable taste for someone who was still in diapers.

I'm not an etiquette expert, but I didn't think children were supposed to register for anything until their wedding. We bought Reyna's precious boy the color-coordinated quilted bowling set that "he" asked for, which he tossed aside upon opening. As we tried to enjoy a piece of gluten-free cowboy cake ("This tastes like paste," my husband whispered to me), we talked with the parents and watched the kids jump in a bounce house.

My husband and I appreciated not being excluded from events just because we didn't have kids. In some cases, these events were the only way we got to see these friends, and we wanted to show support for them and their families. We reasoned that just because our friends had kids, it didn't mean we no longer had interests in common. But at events like Cayden's party, I had to wonder.

A child spread a fistful of frosting onto Reyna's couch cushions, and Stephen's eyes widened. I knew he was thinking of our fabulous couch at home, which cost almost as much as a compact car. My head inevitably started to pound with all the screaming and crying, not to mention the balloon popping and clown horns. I suspected that the clown—as scary as any clown I'd ever seen—was the reason for the kids' crying.

Some time later, Stephen, who was ensconced in a conversation across the room, gave me "that look," the one we'd been honing over the years. At first, our signal was a subtle sequence of winks, which apparently wasn't as subtle as we thought because people thought Stephen was having a seizure. Since then, we've refined that look to a fairly discreet raised eyebrow head-nod gesture.

The signal said two things: (1) Houston, we have a problem, and (2) let's get the hell out of here, immediately.

At once, I kindly excused myself from a rousing conversation about diaper absorbency. I waded through the crowd of adults and sugar-crazed toddlers and finally made my way to my husband.

Right away, I understood the reason for the look. Reyna's husband, Joe, was explaining what Cayden's first solid-food poopie looked like a year and a half ago. Stephen was paralyzed by the horrific descriptions, and who could blame him? I knew what I had to do.

"Joe," I said, "when did you and Reyna have the wainscoting done? It's gorgeous!"

Stephen squeezed my hand in gratitude as Joe launched into an in-depth story about Los Angeles contractors. I smiled to myself. Crisis averted.

Stephen and I had developed an arsenal of stock excuses to help us escape when the party talk inevitably turned to diapers and poopie. At this particular party, we told Reyna and Joe: "Our dogs have been sick, and unless we want to come home to find our house caked with stool, we better get back to walk them."

Reyna and Joe sent us off with sympathetic nods. Nobody ever argued with this one. Nobody asked for additional details to gauge whether we were lying or not. They were happy to let us go. At the time, we didn't even have dogs.

The Condescension

So what if you've got a full-time job, horrible home contractors who are four months behind renovating your only

> "I am sick to death of the type of parents who have this holier-than-thou attitude. People say having a baby changes your life? They've misunderstood the expression. When two people have a child, it changes *their* life. It shouldn't change mine."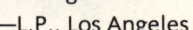
>
> —L.P., Los Angeles

bathroom, unpleasant relatives staying with you indefinitely and treating you like their maid, and your husband asking if you could throw together a dinner party tonight for twelve of his co-workers? If you make the mistake of venting to a mother, you'll most likely hear something like this: "Just wait 'til you have kids. You don't *know* busy."

The three templates for parental condescension are:

1. The "You'll understand when you have kids," or the synonymous "Wait 'til you have kids."
2. The "You don't know _____ [insert noun here—*happiness, love, life, satisfaction*] until you've had a baby."
3. The very rare but deft combination of 1 and 2.

Multiple Choice:

You're at a café waiting for your friend who's bringing her six-month-old baby. She is already a half hour late and hasn't called.

What would you do?

a. Assume she forgot and go on your merry way?
b. Call her and kindly but firmly ask where she is and why she hasn't given a courtesy call?
c. Leave a nasty note with the barista to give to your

friend once she does decide to arrive, long after
you're gone?
   d. Stay and wait and occupy yourself by people watch-
      ing, and try to swallow the anger you feel toward
      this so-called friend?

Unfortunately, I chose *d*. Every time the door opened,
there was a burst of air and light, and in walked someone
else who wasn't the person I was waiting for.

It is a perfect day in Los Angeles. Every day is roughly 68
to 72 degrees and sunny. Lovely. But if you ever remember
asking your parents, "Why can't Christmas be *every* day of
the year?" to which they reply, "It will lose its magic," then
you know why and how this city gets old, fast. I miss variety. I miss seasons. I find myself writing checks in stores
and asking the clerk, "What's the date? Hell, what's the
month and year too, while you're at it?" In other cities,
there are leaves changing, snowflakes falling, buds bloom-
ing, something telling you where you've been and where
you're headed.

Except for two months in the winter, it never rains. I
once thought I heard a clap of thunder, but it turned out to
be a garbage truck barreling down the alley behind my
house.

Geographically, it's kind of a natural oxymoron: the city,
a perpetual construction site, set against the backdrop of
pristine, immutable mountains. My husband and I live at
the bottom of a hill. From one of our windows we can see
the "HO" of the Hollywood sign.

On the sidewalk outside a coffee shop, two men were
shouting at each other. At first glance, I assumed it was a

fight, but then realized they each had a sheet of paper in their hands. They were acting. I saw another fellow who seemed to be college age, setting up for a shot. This happened a lot. I was certain I had appeared in enough student film backgrounds by now to have my own credit list on IMDB.

In a way, living in Los Angeles is like bird watching in an exotic land. So many actors are talking to trees, reciting the two lines over and over that they desperately hope they'll get cast to read.

I once heard that out of all the performers and writers in Los Angeles, only .005 percent actually "make it." I've always wondered what happens to the rest. Does Hollywood have a huge basement that houses all the ones who don't make it? Or do they move away or become accountants eventually or something else more steady?

You can tell by looking at someone's face which part of the journey he or she is on. There's the youthful exuberant hope of ignorance—the fresh-faced ingénue just off the plane from her Alabama college where she won "best actress of the senior class"—versus the faces creased with exhaustion and frustration that broken dreams and the often savage entertainment industry cause, which no cream or serum on the market can cure.

I'm worried that my face now falls into the latter category. I've lived in Los Angeles for almost a decade. I'm a writer, or, rather, an aspiring writer, as I have not yet had a major external success. Everyone is an aspiring writer. You tell someone who doesn't live here that you live in Hollywood, and you hear, "Have I got a movie idea for you. It's my life story, except with a twist. It's a murder mystery and I've been dead the whole time. You should write it!"

My hope has always been that I'd be successful in my career prior to having kids. But I can't control that. I can only work hard, and I do—if it's all about throwing pasta at the wall and seeing what sticks, then I'm wading through a sea of spaghetti.

Forty-five minutes after our initial meeting time, my friend, Sarah, casually walked through the door, pushing her stroller. Even some fake exasperation over her tardiness would have been appreciated at that point. I was about to say something when her baby started to wail. My friend's face contorted. I didn't want to add to her frustration. But what about my frustration? Like I had nothing else going on? Because I don't have a child, it's fine to keep me waiting?

"Where were you?" I asked in my nicest possible tone. Confrontation is no friend of mine. "I was busy!" she said, a little too defensively. "You have no idea how hard it is—just dressing her takes, like, half an hour, then she doesn't want to get into her car seat. You'll understand when you have your own."

There it was—the remark that sent me reeling. If I were better at rebuttals, I might have asked if this was the first time it had taken thirty minutes to dress her, and if not, why wasn't this time delay factored in?

While I bounced her baby on my knee, she asked me, "What's new with you?" to which I expressed my pride over having recently completed a four-hundred-page novel, which took three years to write. To which Sarah responded with another parental whopper, "Wait 'til you have kids. That's the proudest feeling ever."

It's quite possibly true that having a child will eclipse the pleasure and sense of accomplishment I was feeling, having completed my latest book. But why compare the two? I certainly wasn't—I was merely giving a response to her question, sharing my own good news. But if we *were* to compare the two, how about offering one simple word: "Congratulations." I believe that's what I said when she had her baby. For now, at least, this was my baby, and it was gestating for three long, arduous years.

What is at the root of this condescension? Is it just good old-fashioned competition or is it a need to validate or defend our own choices? Is it a catty thing, the female equivalent to "mine is bigger than yours?" I didn't feel threatened when she told me about her child's latest milestone or a fun weekend she had with her family, and I didn't feel the need to justify my existence by comparing my life's work to hers. So why was it necessary to insult my choices in order to boost her own? Was her sense of self so precarious that she thought anyone who chose differently was in some way an affront to her?

Why couldn't we just appreciate the separate paths we'd taken?

"I'm 33 years old with a wonderful husband, happy marriage, great new home, and successful career. We've been trying to get pregnant for a little while with no success, which has led to some disappointment and worry on my part. Add to that the constant pestering, prying, and belly touching that I've been subjected to over these months. Several of the gals I know with kids have decided that what I need to be happy is to be reminded constantly that I *won't* be happy until I produce 2.5 kids and that I better do it soon before it's a nonoption and I'm confined to a life of pointless existence—ha! They need to step off!"

—S.W., Mount Airy, MD

I understood—she had children and they were a ton of work. I respected this, and I was happy for her. But *I* wanted to be afforded the same level of respect and didn't appreciate her downplaying my life, commitments, and choices.

I kept my annoyance over her tardiness to myself, though I beat myself up for it at the time. After that, we didn't talk for a few months. I had no desire to contact her, deciding our friendship was probably over, if not temporarily fractured, because we were at different life stages and she was bent on comparing the two. Then one day she called me out of the blue.

"Wanna meet for lunch tomorrow?" she asked.

Before I could answer, she added, "I promise I'll show up on time."

"Okay," I said. "Sure."

She was waiting for me the next day and had left the baby with a sitter. She was quite repentant, apologizing for her lateness and her behavior at our previous lunch. She told me she had been struggling with her new identity as a mother, was missing her job, and felt a little jealous of women who were doing things besides being what she called "a dairy queen." I was surprised by her admission, but grateful for it.

We talked about both of our identity struggles—hers as a new mother and mine as a new wife who wasn't ready to become a mother and felt as though I'd lost some of my best friends to motherhood. We left the lunch that day stronger friends than we'd ever been, and we remain that way to this day.

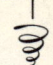

Pre-Partum Pointer: The Holiday Newsletter

Tired of those lengthy, self-absorbed "updates" from distant relatives or friends telling you more than you ever wanted or needed to know about them? ("Little Kitana got a splinter in her index finger. Her first splinter! Can you believe it? And Miller is shaping up to be quite the little drug dealer—four sales in one week!")

Then fight back by sending out one of your own!

If you're single, list every doctor's appointment you had that year, and report the blood, cholesterol, and urinalysis results with pride!

If you're married with no kids, discuss the complicated office politics at your job and then describe in great detail each of the tricks your dog/cat/parakeet can do.

If you've got kids, take the newsletter to a whole new level by mentioning them only in passing and making it all about you, obnoxiously so. "We went to Aspen then to India and then to Tuscany where we spent several weeks sipping wine in its tranquil hills. I think the kids came with us on that last one, but I'm not 100 percent sure. We were really drunk."

Practice

Before we got married, Stephen and I agreed we'd get a dog before starting a family, thinking this would be the perfect internship in parenthood. Just after our first Christmas as a married couple, we found our intern: a tiny pup in a picture on a website.

Before we left to pick up the puppy, we called my parents to tell them of our impending addition.

"Hey mom," I said.

Stephen got on the phone as well. I cleared my throat. "Stephen and I just wanted to tell you—"

My mother stopped me, barely covering the phone with her hand, and screamed, "RICK! Get on the phone! Carrie and Stephen have an announcement! THIS IS IT!"

"Oh no no no" I yelled through the phone. "Um, mom? It's not that—"

My dad got on the phone. He was giddy with excitement: "Geezie? What do you have to tell us?"

He and my mom seemed so happy. I felt terrible that our news wasn't going to live up to their expectations.

"Oh, um, we're just . . . we're going to get a dog today."

Silence.

"A little puppy," I said, thinking the cute factor might help cushion the blow.

More silence.

"It's a beagle!" my husband said, appealing to their love of the breed.

Finally, they both started talking simultaneously, sounding like chickens clucking around feed, "Oh! Huh! Neat! What? Okay! Great! Congrats!" barely able to contain their surprise and disappointment.

We drove up to a house in the snowy San Gabriel Mountains and were greeted by the breeder, a woman who stood pitched forward, either because of back trouble or because of the gravitational pull of her enormous breasts. When we entered her home, we noticed that beagles were *everywhere:* old ones, young ones, beagle portraits, beagle figurines, beagle light-switch covers, beagle tapestries, and beagle Kleenex cozies. And in the corner, in an otherwise empty plastic baby pool, one tiny beagle head popped up, trying to get a good look at us. We went over and kneeled beside him.

He had the requisite Cro-Magnon puppy head, complete with prominent brow bone, almost like an awning of fur over his eyes. His fur was so black it was practically blue, like an oil slick or Superman's hair. He stared up at me with his big light gray eyes, such a piercing contrast against the rest of him. "Are you my mother?" his gaze asked. Just like that, it was love. And then he took a dump that can only be described as monumentally huge. My husband, of course, marveled at how much could come out of a five-pound creature. "He's a freakin' Play-Doh factory!" he said, with what sounded like pride. Men. A trained eye might have questioned the breeder, after this tiny pup pooped all over the space in which he slept. If we'd done our homework, we might have suspected the dog had worms or some worse parasite, but we didn't know that at the time. We thought the shit storm was, well, kismet. He had, after all, a very strong reaction when he first saw us, as did we.

We liked the name Beauregard for a dog and thought it was ostentatious yet regal, kitschy. But as I stared at the puppy looking up at me from the palm of my hand—his hummingbird-like energy, the fact his whole body wagged—I knew the joke wouldn't sustain itself. The name was far too long and far too big for such a tiny dude. So we shortened his name to the more playful, accessible "Bowie."

That night, once we were home, the new surroundings proved an overload for our little pup. We put him in his crate at bedtime, but he looked at me with those big, droopy eyes and his long face while letting out a heart-breaking wail that sounded like he was being flayed.

Against my better judgment, I took Bowie out and cuddled with him in our bed. He stopped whining, but his gurgles and grunts and readjustments kept me awake. Three heartbeats in a bed that used to house only two felt risky. While sleeping, he had a bout of the hiccups that rattled his whole body like little thunderstorms. He had a nursing dream where his paws cupped and uncupped, and his mouth made this delicious sucking sound. With the symphony of sounds, I couldn't sleep: I was both fascinated and scared to death. What if he fell out of bed? What if I rolled over and crushed him?

My bigger concern should have been, what if he poops again? But before I had a chance to worry about it, he was squatting in our bed, the pungent odor waking us from our fitful sleeps. There was diarrhea everywhere—on the comforter, blanket, sheets, and mattress, which even soaked down into the mattress padding.

We spent the rest of the first night of our parenting internship dozing in our living room—I was on the couch and Stephen was curled up on the loveseat. In the middle of the night, Bowie wriggled off my chest and into my armpit. After he tired of that location, he wriggled again. In a split second I recognized it, but a split second too late: he was already rolling off the couch. I watched in slow motion, paralyzed, as he careened to the unforgiving living room floor. I don't know exactly what he landed on—his tiny birdlike rib cage, his cute already scrunched face, or his diamond-encrusted back. I cradled him on the floor and tested all his bones with my fingers, watched him walk, and looked for limps, and then I summarily beat myself up for being the worst mother of all time.

Delirious from lack of sleep, I started laughing and crying at the same time. Stephen opened his eyes and looked at me across our living room. He said in a monotone voice, "What have we done? This is a fucking nightmare."

I laughed and cried harder. We were exhausted. Our house smelled like dog poop. And this was only the first night!

"Does the breeder have a return policy?" he asked, laughing but also clearly contemplating it. I, too, was filled with regret and I hated myself for it. What kind of mother would I be if I couldn't even handle a little puppy?

"What are we going to do if we have a difficult kid? We wouldn't give him up, would we?" I asked Stephen. Part of me was proving a point, but part of me was really asking. Stephen drifted back to sleep while I lay awake feeling utterly incompetent, with my new, furry obligation snoring on my chest.

One thing was certain: we were a long way off from having kids.

CHAPTER THREE

Baby Lust

Now the thing about having a baby—and I can't be the first person to have noticed this—is that thereafter you have it.

—JEAN KERR

Shortly after Christmas, one of my closest girlfriends and I had dinner. Kay was aglow with good news—she had just sold her first screenplay. We cheered and toasted to her success. She told me she would also be producing the project—right around the time she was producing another project: a baby! I sat in stunned silence for five seconds that felt like five minutes. Had I heard her correctly? Were she and her husband even trying for a baby?

"Roy's over the moon!" she said and beamed.

It was hard to imagine her husband, Roy, doing anything besides hunching over a video game in their living room. To be fair, I'd only met him a handful of times. They'd only been married a few months, and their wedding was just six weeks after they went on their first date.

45

When Kay met Roy, she was wild and funny and wore very convincing knockoffs of the kinds of shoes you only see on *Sex and the City*. Kay would typically fall fast and hard for a guy and then forget all about him a month later. There was always neediness to her dating, as if she relied on these men to define her. She grew up thinking she was a problem that needed solving. Those of us close to her always believed she was perfect the way she was.

Then Roy came on the scene, a painter and part-time acoustic guitarist whom she met at a mutual friend's party. She fell for him, fast; she stopped wearing high heels because they felt like they were "holding her feet prisoner," and she invited us to a singalong that turned out to be their surprise wedding. "Bring an instrument, your voice, and an open mind!" the Evite had said.

"Is this a singalong or an orgy?" another one of our friends asked.

Once I collected myself, I screamed my surprise and delight about my friend's upcoming "productions."

"When it rains it pours, right?" she said. "It's an embarrassment of riches!"

Immediately, I was reminded of that great exchange in *Broadcast News* when William Hurt asks Albert Brooks, "What do you do when your real life exceeds your dreams?" to which Brooks replies, "You keep it to yourself." This is how I feel about the phrase "an embarrassment of riches," but don't get me wrong, I love Kay and wish her happiness. I don't care how evolved or at peace you are—even Mother Theresa or Gandhi at least once in their lives felt a little jealous of those with great luck. It draws out my abundance issues, making me feel as though there's only so much happy to go around, and one person's success is another's failure. Intellectually, I know that's not true, but irrationally, I get that feeling sometimes. I'm not proud of it but I do. I am also envious of Kay's self-confidence, to take this leap into parenthood so boldly, jumping in with both feet.

I felt something else too. Loneliness. This was my last married friend to embark on the wonders of childbearing. In the past, we'd lament together about how many of our mutual friends and acquaintances had turned into "momzillas" almost overnight.

Now she was joining the club. Not that she would ever become a momzilla—she was the most organized and capable woman I've known. But I still felt like I was losing a friend, not gaining another friend with a baby.

The temptation to succumb to baby lust and to start trying for a child of my own was rarely stronger than in situations like this one, when friends announced they were pregnant. I felt 75 percent ready to start a family immediately, but knew I needed to be closer to 100 percent, lest I regret or resent.

Kay and I had a good night after that, chatting away about her two upcoming productions, but I was already aware that the night was probably one of the last of its kind for a while.

I raised my glass to my friend one more time, trying to swallow the bittersweetness that was caught in my throat.

The Pitter-Patter

I love babies. I love their smell, their little fingers and toes, their baby babble, their smiles, the looks on their faces when they're taking in the world. I'm crazy about kids. This rarely waivers. I'm not so crazy about some of their parents, but we'll get to that later.

We've all had those experiences where the kid was so cute your teeth hurt. For me, it was when a three-year-old who I was babysitting for told his first joke. He was so tickled with the fact that he'd made it up and delivered the punch line that he laughed himself silly. It was a moment I'll never forget.

When I was six years old, I'd swaddle my dolls the way I had seen my mother swaddle my baby brother and then I'd baby dance all over the house with my doll on my shoulder, patting her back ever so gently and singing her songs I'd make up as I'd go along. When I was nine and my friends were stuffing their bras, I was padding my belly and then walking around the neighborhood, pushing a stroller with my dolls in it.

In my twenties, I ended some of my most serious relationships because the guy either didn't want to settle down to have babies or wanted to commit but didn't want to have babies or wanted them but wouldn't have made a good dad to any future kids. Motherhood was the only job I ever wanted.

Pre-Partum Pointer: Beware of Scary Baby Lust

Expressions of endearment about your friends' adorable munchkins that may sound good in your head but don't out loud:

- Your kids are so cute I could eat them with a spoon!
- They're so cute I just wanna squeeze them like a tube of toothpaste!
- They're so cute I want to bite them. Not 'til they bleed, just gnawing, really. I wouldn't break the skin, I promise.
- I totally understand kidnapping now!

I changed majors in college almost every semester and career paths often, but I've always wanted to raise a family.

I was nearly 27 when I met Stephen. I knew he was the man for me based on many wonderful qualities. But the moment I knew I wanted to marry him was on our second date, when he told me a story about his two beloved nephews and the way they were so different from one another and would "direct" Stephen's made-up stories according to their different personalities. "Eli's like a development executive when he's asking for his story, 'I want drama, and action, a dragon, and a happy ending. Go!'"

Stephen told the story with such love and humor, with a clear understanding of children and human nature, and I knew at that moment that I couldn't wait to have kids with this man.

"We are madly in love, have been together for 6 years and married for 3 years. My husband is 40 and I am 35. The natural progression both biologically and socially would be to procreate. There are times when I see a child and am consumed with fascination, joy, and appreciation for this beautiful creation, but it seems way too exhausting. I like the freedom that we have. It might seem selfish, but sometimes I think it's selfish to bring a little clone of yourself into the world. I know that we'd be excellent, nurturing parents. But is that enough? Is that reason enough to bring a child into this world? Most of the time I don't think so. Maybe we're overthinking it, though I'm not sure there is such a thing, especially in today's screwed-up world. I wish other couples would give it more thought before just doing what they think they're supposed to or what everyone around them is doing."

—E.S., Denver, CO

And yet, a year and a half later, we were still waiting. I suppose the security of our marriage combined with our jobs and travels took over. We'd been thoroughly enjoying each other's company. We'd even developed our own little language.

Even though we had decided to wait to have kids, sometimes it felt like the universe was trying to tell us something. As we were pulling into our driveway after our first wedding anniversary dinner, Stephen and I saw a little boy crying in the middle of the street in front of our house. We pulled over and ran up to him.

Of course, I, with my flair for the dramatic, immediately thought about baby Moses in the reeds of the riverbank.

We knelt on either side of him. He wasn't speaking English and couldn't have been more than four years old. He wore a pajama set, the pants twisted around his trunk and legs. The shirt had a silk-screened baseball mitt graphic and said "Major League Baseball USA!"—the sort of exuberant, patriotic exclamation only found on clothes not made in the USA.

Stephen spoke French to him and translated for me. "He had a fight with his mama," Stephen told me. "Where does your mama live?" he asked the boy in French. The little boy tugged on my hand and then put both arms in the air, the international sign for "pick me up." I lifted him and held him and rubbed his back. Suddenly, there was no language barrier between us—he was scared and upset, and I was trying to comfort him and make it all okay.

The three of us went from house to house, knocking on doors. "It's okay, buddy, we'll find her," Stephen said to him. In my head, though, I was already wondering if we would and, if we didn't, I was mentally converting my den into his bedroom. Blue's a little overdone. Maybe try sailboats or—duh!—baseball. Or maybe something soft and soothing, like clouds, like the kid's room in *Kramer vs. Kramer*. I'd always loved that room. When he grew up a little more and asked about how we came to be his parents, we'd tell him he was meant to be our little boy (leaving out the clunky detail that "we found you on our lawn"), and say the precious explanation of adoption, "You were born in my heart."

Stephen knocked on every door until we found the mother—a weary-looking woman with a baby on each hip. It was unclear whether she'd even noticed that her son was gone. We put him down and he ran to her, crying and hugging her legs. We explained where we found him, and the mother knelt down and kissed the top of his head. She looked at us and said "merci" half a dozen times.

As stressed out and exhausted as she seemed, in that moment, more than anything, I wanted to be her. I wanted to hug the little boy and read him a bedtime story and take care of him as if he were my own.

Some people confuse baby lust with societal pressure. Everyone knows at least one of those couples who clearly has a case of the "now what's." After the wedding and the honeymoon, they realize it is just the two of them and that feeling of "now what?" sneaks up. The wedding planning's over and the party's done. Now they're left with—each other. This is when lots of couples decide to get pregnant. The first year of marriage is the hardest, for a reason: it's a period of substantial adjustment to each other's lifestyles, habits, and quirks and a time to negotiate your now combined finances and holidays with in-laws.

It seems kind of selfish or unprepared to bring children

The Now What's

Factoid:

    BabyCenter.com asked nearly 60,000 people how long they had been in their relationships prior to getting pregnant with their first child. The results showed that 15% reported less than a year, 17% said between 1–2 years, 24% said between 2–4 years, and 19% said between 4–6 years.

Opinionoid:

    You should wait at least until your wedding pictures are back from the printers before trying to conceive. Why not forge as strong a bond as possible before adding kids to the mix? Go ahead, order your wedding photos and wait the six months or so for them to arrive, all shiny and frame ready. Meanwhile, cuddle up with your spouse and plan a trip together.

---

into the world when you or your relationship aren't quite ready—sort of like living in Kansas without a tornado cellar.

My husband and I hadn't suffered from the now what's—despite my bouts of baby lust here and there—largely because we were terrified about taking that next step. Meanwhile, some friends of mine never gave themselves a chance even to consider the next step. They just jumped right in. In a moment of unguarded honesty, Reyna once mentioned that she "wished" she'd had a chance to be scared before she got pregnant because now she's scared retrospectively. "I worry about everything," she told me. "I know that's a part of parenting, but not like

> "A baby can't fix a thing. If anything, having our son has brought my husband and me further apart. We're so tired all the time and we've got different ideas about how to raise him. Even though he's only three, he pits us against each other, whether he's aware of it or not. That's not something I expected—that having a kid would make any little problems we had flair up instead of putting them on the back burner more."
> —Anonymous, Worcester, MA

this. I stand over Cayden and watch him sleep for at least an hour every night. I'm on drugs for anxiety. This isn't normal. If I'd known I'd feel this way, I'd have waited longer to have a baby. And I'll bet I wouldn't be *quite* as anxious as I am now."

When Reyna was pregnant—and she was the first to admit this—she spent most of her pregnancy decorating the baby's nursery. Instead of preparing herself for motherhood, she gutted the nursery, added built-in shelves, ordered a custom crib, and had the carpet and drapes flown in from France. It's a gorgeous nursery, but the parenting books on the beautiful built-in shelves still have uncracked bindings.

> "A friend of mine has admitted that she's not really enjoying being a mom. She thought it might grow on her, but it hasn't. Yet every couple of years, she's pregnant again. I feel like that's so unfair to the kids she keeps on having because she doesn't enjoy raising them and it shows. She's not exactly great at it, yet for whatever reasons, she keeps on popping them out."
> —J.M., St. Louis, MO

I can't necessarily blame her. Once you become en-sconced in the world of "baby," it's probably easy to forget that you're about to become a parent when you can fall in love with baby "stuff" instead.

Buy Buy Baby

A little over a year into our marriage, I was surrounded by pregnant women. If they weren't friends or relatives, they were celebrities on TV. They were everywhere. I attended approximately two baby showers or brisses a month. And when I wasn't at the showers personalizing onesies with pastel paints, I was scrolling down friends' gift registries and settling on a Boppy, chipping in on a Bugaboo, or find-ing out the latest recall information about a Bumbo.

I love baby stuff. Who doesn't? I've always enjoyed shop-ping for friends and acquaintances, but I don't think I real-ized how severe my own case of baby lust was until I spent an evening scrolling through my friend Kay's online baby registry.

It started innocently enough: After I purchased a gift on her registry (a fabulous car seat that's ideal for air travel because it has a telescoping handle and wheels that turn it into a stroller), I idly browsed the website, clicking on dif-ferent categories such as diaper supplies, cribs, feeding supplies, and gear.

There was a gorgeous baby swing with white tulle draped around it and a lamp on top with star cutouts that, according to the product description, projected stars all over the room, while baby swung to sleep. Why didn't they make these sorts of items in adult size? I imagined myself watching my perfect newborn fall asleep in a swing like that, stars thrown all over the walls of the perfect nursery. I clicked on the description and noticed some previous users had rated the swing already. How helpful! Comments like "Pretty swing but it broke." "Loud motor." "Eats through batteries too fast." Well, what did they know?

My reflexes took over. I clicked a button and poof—the Starlight Swing was in my online shopping cart. Once I realized what I had done, I immediately deleted it. I was not going to purchase a $99 swing for a baby who didn't even exist yet! So I filed it in my long-term memory that the swing, while pretty, needed a lot of batteries.

I continued clicking through the website, reading and learning about all sorts of other products. I was a sponge, sopping up as much baby information as possible. And every bit of new information was a revelation and led me to another product, and another:

Images in vivid colors and bold black-and-white stimulate early visual tracking!

Infants need tummy time!

Glass bottles that are vented give babies less gas bubbles!

Toys that don't require batteries and are "kid-powered" are ways to encourage active, not passive, thinking in children!

Glass bottles are free of Bisphenol-A! I had no idea what Bisphenol-A was, but did I want my precious fictitious babies ingesting it? Hell no!

I wrote myself a post-it that said, "Bisphenol-A is BAD," to remember when I start having kids, as my memory has never been very reliable. It could hold onto the Starlight Swing, but not much more than that. I couldn't find any place to stick the post-it, as my desk looks like the inside of a dumpster. There were notes and articles and packets and books I'd been meaning to read for the last two years and New Years' resolution lists from 2001 among piles organized in a way that once made sense to me. The post-it about Bisphenol-A was as good as lost.

If only I could create a wish list of sorts right there on the baby store's website of things I wanted to remember to get whenever it became my turn!

And then I wondered: Why couldn't I make a sort of fake registry, one that I could update on my own?

I scrolled down the many baby-store registries, and some of the due dates listed were impossible: 1/1/11. That's a mighty long gestation period. And the dates were under names like Yogi Berra, Daffy Duck, and Mickey Mouse. So, clearly, other people had done what I was considering doing. What was the harm in creating a tiny list for my tiny, unborn children under another name? Obviously I didn't expect to receive the gifts (at least not until I changed it over to my own name, someday), but that wasn't the point. The point was to remember what these great products were and to update them as trends and research changed.

I typed in a fake name, based on a childhood pet and the street I grew up on. Sure enough, it sounded like a porn star's name. I entered a date that was approximately nine months away. My face burned, as it did when I was doing something sneaky. But who was going to catch me? The baby store web police? Was Big Baby watching?

In under a minute, my registry was set and ready. "Add items now!" it beckoned.

Twist my arm, why don't you.

I jumped right into the educational and developmental toys category because there's never been anything more important than making sure my imaginary kids develop their imaginations as much as possible. I clicked on rattles and pull toys and dolls that promised to reward curiosity and build cognitive skills or that taught eye-hand coordination, tactile and fine motor skills, and shape and color recognition. How could I say no? I wanted the best for my children! Who doesn't?

I added them all to my registry.

Under "related products," there was a bouncy ball that won the iParenting media award in 2007! I didn't know what the iParenting award was, but how could I pass that up? "Add."

I read about something called the fourth trimester, in which newborns like to be swaddled, as it makes them feel as contained as they were in the womb. I chose a few blankets in gender-neutral colors: a sunny light yellow and another in serene sage green, in case one was in the wash. "Add, add."

And the website, always so helpful, reminded me not to forget about the white noise machine that simulates sounds from mommy's womb. "Add."

No-scratch mittens are a must!

Shampoo rinse cup!

Tummy-time playmats!

No-skid fish stickers for the bottom of the bathtub!

Breast cream!

Standard Pack 'n Play that grows with baby over time!

Small Pack 'n Play for trips to Grandma's house!

Pacifiers!

Thermometer pacifiers!

Burp pads, travel systems, baby monitors, oh my!

It felt as if I were going on a shopping spree without having to move or spend a cent. At midnight, three hours after I began, my fake registry had 117 items on it.

Many things occurred to me as I looked at this list on my computer, the first being that I had completely lost my mind.

"I think it's sweet," my therapist said, a week later.

"Don't patronize me," I told him. "I know I should be locked up or heavily medicated or both."

He wrote something on his notepad.

"Is that a prescription?" I asked, hopefully.

"No, Carrie. I think it's sweet that you're already so interested in giving your unborn children the best you can. You'll certainly be prepared!"

"I appreciate your kindness, but you can be straight with me. On the spectrum of crazy, what am I? A 9? 10?"

"Look," he said, "it would be an entirely different situation if you were actually purchasing these items. Then you'd be a hoarder or a shopaholic or both. But this is just a wish list of sorts, right?"

"Of course!" I said. "Or more of a memory device for what I might need whenever the time comes. And it's my weird way of blowing off steam. It's like my equivalent to a normal person's World of Warcraft habit. Still, I hate the fact I know that the woman walking past me with her baby this morning was doing so with Graco's Snugride Safeseat carrier (#1 car seat in 2007's crash tests) in the playful, fun, gender-neutral Safari Friends pattern with French Roast trim, atop Baby Trend's $59 Snap 'N Go stroller frame. I'm like the Rain Man of baby gear. 'Yes, definitely Baby Einstein, definitely Baby Einstein. . . . Dad lets me drive my Cozy Push and Ride by Little Tikes slowly in the driveway.' "

He laughed, then put his notepad down.

"Listen," he said. "I actually have another patient who's looking for a good bouncer/swing combo. Her kid's colicky. Any recommendations?"

"Very funny," I said. "I'm laughing on the inside."

"No, I mean it. Any thoughts?"

I leaned forward and immediately became flushed with excitement. I salivated a little. "Actually, there are only a few combos on the market, but they're really the smartest buy. They're called three-in-ones and have settings that can make them bounce in a stationary setting, vibrate, or turn into a swing. This way, you don't need to buy a separate bouncer and swing. Brilliant, right?"

He smiled, but it felt like he was pitying me. "Oh, Carrie," he said.

"What?" I asked. "Oh crap. I'm so far gone that I'm not even on the spectrum of crazy?"

"No," he said. "Our time's up."

Was I craving an actual baby or just their things? I decided that having baby lust in a kid's store, whether it's clothing, toys, furniture, or accessories, can't count as a legitimate desire to have children. After all, when a baby's screaming at three in the morning, the adorable onesie he's crapping all over won't mean a whole lot.

A single girlfriend of mine has called, on occasion, and sung into the phone, "I want to have a baby so badly!"

"Did you just come from Half-Pint?" I always ask.

"How'd you know?"

Half-Pint is her favorite children's clothing store in Los Angeles. I do not go anymore because I am too tempted to buy one of everything. The last time I went, I fell in love with a baby wetsuit and matching pair of baby-sized swimming flippers. When you really think about it, it makes no sense and is probably, in fact, terribly dangerous for a kid to be toddling around in flippers especially near water. But when shopping under the influence of baby stores (or SUI), common sense flies out the window, and this weird baby adrenaline (which is produced, I imagine, by the ovaries) takes over and convinces me I must have a set of baby flippers in every color. Luckily, I refrain.

Another place where I always have difficulty controlling myself is in the children's sections at bookstores. I love the covers and the artwork, and I like imagining which books my kids and I will read together. Some are classics I remember loving when I was a child (*Corduroy the Bear*, *The Giving Tree*, *Where the Wild Things Are*) and others are new and adorable (*Don't Let the Pigeon Drive the Bus*, *Guess How Much I Love You*, *If You Give a Moose a Muffin*). I could spend the entire day wandering this section. I haven't mainly because a bookstore employee always asks if I need help finding anything. I say, "Nah, just browsing." That employee inevitably follows up with, "What age child are you browsing for?"

I'm always tempted to say, "Um, 27?" but instead I admit, "No child in particular."

While I may refrain from baby shopping for my own nonexistent baby in my everyday life, shopping for my friends' babies is a welcome excuse to enter these baby palaces and actually purchase something. Walking through the aisles of Babies "R" Us with a friend's registry in hand, I admired her choices: the beautiful sage toile playard, the sweet Winnie the Pooh mobile, and the ergonomic jogging stroller whose tires looked more durable than my SUVs. I mentally noted what items to add to my fake online registry once I got home.

For a few minutes in this baby wonderland, I slipped into a pretty, pastel place where I was holding my very own pink-faced newborn, his/her (my dreams never specify gender) tiny hand wrapped around my index finger. In this fantasy, I was the picture of a composed, natural mother: my lips wearing subtle nude Nars lipstick, my cheekbones lightly shaded and my long natural hair cascading in perfect curls down my shoulders, gently grazing Baby's soft cheek as I swaddled him/her in the precious 360 thread count sage toile blanket (that came with the matching playard, of course). In this reverie I had already lost the baby weight and all my parts had healed seamlessly. Nurses say mine is the most beautiful baby they've ever seen, and then I blush. "You say that to all the new mothers, I'm sure."

"No, we really don't," they say—

"I WANT THE DOLLY!!!!" A three year old's temper tantrum snapped me back to reality in the aisles of Babies "R" Us. The child shoved the mother and then writhed on the floor. The mother looked like she was contemplating just leaving the kid in the store. My head started throbbing instantly, my daydream shattered. I grabbed a BabyBjörn, paid, and ran out.

I don't blame the screaming child for my rude awakening. I blame *People* magazine. I've gotten most of my false visions from its sumptuous but unrealistic celebrity baby spreads. *People* has made pregnancy and childbearing look glamorous and easy. Not so, say many close friends of mine. There's gas and bloating and swollen feet and cankles and spit-up, and you forget to brush your teeth for days at a time.

Yet many of us look at the glossy pages of *People* and forget about all the hard stuff. We're just so tickled to be invited into JLo's or Brangelina's nurseries. We revel in the baby love in the photos, but what we really want is the fantasy of their lifestyle. I want JLo's nursery, complete with the cream and mocha walls and dupioni silk drapes that probably, alone, cost more than my house. I want a staff of sixty to anticipate my needs and wait on me hand and foot. I want the fancy $3,000 Silver Cross pram, and I wouldn't mind cashmere sweater sets like the ones the babies were wearing, if they came in my size.

We want to look like Jennifer and Angelina a month after giving birth, with their perfect caramel curls and muted makeup and designer gowns, instead of like a puffy, waddling, stitched-together mess of leaky fluids. This fantasy is the new equivalent to comparing ourselves to Photoshopped models in magazines the way we did when we were seventeen. Instead of comparing ourselves to impossible ideals of beauty, we compare ourselves to impossible ideals of motherhood.

The stars make it look simple. Of course a celebrity appears surprisingly well rested for the parent of one-month-

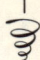

Parent Peeve: Celebration Rings

If an additional gift of jewelry is necessary, perhaps you shouldn't be having a baby. Isn't the child gift enough?

old twins! Because her makeup artist spends half a day perfecting that look and odds are the movie star's not the one rolling out of bed and shlepping back and forth in the middle of the night for feedings.

These magazines fly off the shelves, but what are we really buying into?

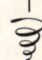

Quiz Yourself!

Kids' product brand or porn movie title?

1. Dream on Me
2. Joovy Big Caboose (stand-on tandem)
3. Floppy Products
4. Blowfish
5. Baby Sac
6. Badger Basket
7. Ima Rose-N-Bloom
8. Dana Undies

Answers: Believe it or not, all these are kids products or brand names or both.

Factoid:

In a poll, 65,000 people were asked if they would have done anything differently before having kids: 65 percent said yes, they would have done some things differently. Of those, 25 percent wished they had paid off more debt and become more financially secure, 21 percent wished they'd had more fun (which included travel, parties, and movies), and 18 percent wished they had completed their educations.

—BabyCenter.com

Pregnancy Propaganda

My gynecologist was checking under the hood. While she did so, she talked about restaurants she and her husband liked in the area. I inserted a few well-placed uh-huhs and reallys, but personally, I've never loved making chitchat while a lady doctor's all up in my grill, much less chitchat about food. I've always felt like we should just accept that it's an awkward situation and remain silent out of respect.

I let my mind drift outside the sterile doctor's office, to a more pleasant place. I imagined myself on a beach, the waves lapping on the shore, seagulls cackling. A shirtless Brad Pitt walked up with one of his kids in tow. I wished the kid would leave so I could be alone with Brad, but it was one of the adopted ones, and he had separation anxiety. Even my daydreams have obstacles. I asked him how Angelina was. He said it wasn't working out between them because she was too beautiful. I nodded. I understood.

Then Brad said, "You're almost 30 now, right?"

All too quickly, I was back on the cold examination table.

"No," I said to my doctor. "I turn 30 in eight months." I clung to those eight months.

"And you and your husband want to have kids?"

I nodded, then remembered she couldn't see me. "Yep."

"When are you thinking about trying?"

What did she want me to do? Give her a date? "A year?" I said.

Her eyebrows raised.

"You think less?" I asked, trying to gauge her reaction.

"How long have you been married, Carrie?"

"Two years," I said.

"Everything's going okay?"

"Everything's great!" I said. What was she, my shrink?

"You know, you're in good health. If you're planning on it, I recommend you do it sooner rather than later. Every year that goes by, you have less egg follicles."

Like I wasn't aware of that.

I couldn't help but think my doctor should have known better than to pressure patients into having kids before they were ready.

The walls of the exam room were covered with framed, soft-focus pictures of a beautiful, glowing pregnant woman, a beautiful glowing new mother holding her perfect bundle of joy, a glowing husband and wife playing with their perfect cherub. Were these pictures advertising pregnancy and child rearing? And why? Were the numbers low?

Everywhere I look today, there's another pregnancy bump popping up! There's that crazy woman who has eighteen kids! Should there perhaps be a "Quality over Quantity" law? For all we know, she's overpopulating our planet with future bank robbers and murderers because she is too busy getting knocked up to pay attention to her kids eating paste and setting the dog on fire.

As I left the doctor's office, a very pregnant woman waddled out in front of me, holding her three-year-old daughter's hand.

"Press the button, Hailey," the mom said, then turned and winked at me, like "check this out, my kid's about to do something unbelievably cute."

The little girl *was* very cute. But she wasn't pressing the elevator's down button. She just stood there, picking at her glittery nail polish.

"Hailey, press the button," the mother repeated.

The entire lobby of the OB-GYN office was covered with similar photos to those in the exam room—it was like pregnancy propaganda. They must have been on sale in bulk. I could tell that the models who posed for the pictures weren't even considering getting pregnant at the time, let alone actually pregnant. I had heard from all my girlfriends who'd had babies that the real-life experience wasn't quite as soft-focused and dreamy. For one thing, the women in the photos weren't retaining so much water that their fingers looked like sausages. Where was the soft-focus photo depicting a woman who peed a little bit every time she sneezed or laughed? Do you know what an episiotomy is? I do, and it doesn't sound pretty.

Weren't these photos dangerous? They were setting it up so that if you didn't feel exactly like that—all soft-focus, dreamy, and pastelly—right away you felt as though something was wrong with you. Did that, perhaps, contribute to some cases of post-partum depression?

Little Hailey still hadn't pressed the down button to call for the elevator. "Okay, Hale, Mama's gonna do it then," the mom said and, thankfully, started to point at the button.

"NOoOOoOOooo!" the little girl screamed. "I wanna do it. You said I could do it!"

"When things don't go according to the 'best-case scenarios' described in all the countless books and magazines because of things quite out of your control (e.g., emergency c-section, inability to produce breast milk), it leaves you feeling like there is already a ding against you."

—L.I., Portland, OR

"Okay," the mom said. "Then press the button. Last chance, sweetheart."

The child didn't press the damn button. And mom started trying to coax her again.

I pressed the button. The mother looked at me, stunned.

"Sorry," I said. "I've got someplace to be." Never mind the fact that the place I had to be was in a hot bath, saying "Calgon, take me away!" For all she knew, I was a surgeon and had just been called to emergency surgery but wouldn't make it in time because darling Hailey was given the enormous responsibility of pressing the button. Once the three of us were in the elevator car, Hailey carried on, screaming about how she wanted to press the button.

The elevator car was lined with even more happy baby photos. I wished I could have taken a picture of this little elevator scene, as it was more realistic. I was starting to wonder if there was a not-so-subtle agenda, reinforced on multiple levels, to subdue women by romanticizing pregnancy and motherhood. What about all those movies in which the woman finally felt complete once she had gotten "her baby" and the commercials that enticed you with their heartstring-tugging ads so that if any woman didn't want to have a baby, or didn't enjoy the thought of child rearing, she knew to keep her mouth shut for fear of being branded a bad woman? Celebrity magazines had played into this propaganda. If a new mother didn't feel as elated as JLo purported to be or hadn't snapped back into shape as fast as Christina Aguilera, she felt like there was something wrong with her. Perhaps there should be disclaimers at the bottom of blissful baby commercials and magazine spreads, much like the ones they put at the bottom of weight loss ads: "Results Not Typical."

Delusting

When precious baby items and pristine images of motherhood surround you, it's easy to forget that there will be an actual baby to take care of. Over the years, to curb my own baby lust, I've thought of some ways to counteract it and give myself a reality check.

Pre-Partum Pointer: Best Birth Control Methods Not on the Market

- Plant a garden and try not to kill it.
- Babysit.
- Spend 10 minutes with a colicky baby.
- Take our puppy for a week. (Please.)

Plant a Garden and Try to Keep It Alive

In ninth grade, we had to walk around with a potted plant all day long for a week to simulate, I supposed, the effects of teen parenthood and the crushing responsibility it brings. Kind of ridiculous when you thought about it, as a plant made no noise and didn't go doodie in its pot and require changing, but whatever. I put a pretty blue ribbon around him (for some reason I decided my plant was a boy). I named him Ralph J. Friedman and fashioned a sling in which to carry him. I stopped short of sending out birth announcements. In all my obsessive loving of him, I forgot to water the little guy and he died under my care, his leaves brown and crispy. More than a little disconcerting and proof, I suppose, that love just wasn't enough.

Fifteen years later and much closer to parenthood than back then, I'm finding I still don't have the magic touch when it comes to plant life. I've sowed numerous vegetable gardens—chives, parsley, tomatoes, salad greens—and for about a week, after the seeds have germinated, I'm on cloud nine, feeling like the environmentalist of the year, adding more green to this earth and more oxygen to my home. But as fast as my pride over the plants moves in, so does the prompt desiccation of said plants. It's as if they can sense my confidence and immediately wilt, becoming mere sleeper cells for aphids and fruit flies.

I even managed to screw up a Zen garden. That took real skill. Our new pup seemed to think the sand was his personal restroom. There was nothing peaceful or Zen about that.

My biggest problem with plant care is that I have yet to find the delicate balance between nourishing the plants and leaving them alone. They die either of starvation or of overwatering. I figure this care will make them grow faster and stronger, but it ends up killing them—an apt metaphor for my biggest fears about parenting.

Creative Concept: The RealCare® Baby

Realityworks, a company based in the Midwest, created The RealCare® Baby infant simulator. Schools across the country are now using these computer-tracked dolls to prevent teen pregnancy, encourage abstinence, and educate future parents and caregivers. Based on the schedules of 15 real infants, these dolls cry when they need anything—to be burped, fed, rocked, or changed—and will cry until that particular need is met. Sensors on their body detect abuse and are programmed to respond only to its "parent."

Babysit

While I love kids, I know they're a lot of work. I worked in an after-school program, substitute-taught first grade, and nannied and babysat since I was eleven years old. I realize none of those are motherhood, but they're probably as close as you can get without having kids of your own.

For all those years, I was just having fun because working with children was my favorite way to spend time. Now I see it was also invaluable on-the-job training. But did all that experience ruin me in some ways for the future? Am I that much more reluctant because I have an inkling of how much work and toil is involved?

Spend Ten Minutes with a Colicky Baby

In my day (yes, I'm officially a thousand), there weren't these fancy swings that constantly ran and had vibration modes to lull your baby. Now you can put a colicky baby in one of those puppies, flip on the switch, and enjoy at least a little quiet time, maybe even sneak in a quick shower. Back in my babysitting days, the swings had noisy, rusty crank handles that needed rewinding every five minutes. And if you didn't have a swing or bouncer, you had to hold the baby while constantly moving. One memorable night of babysitting, I did the baby dance for five hours; that's five hours straight of this little darling screaming his head off in my ear. By the end of that impossibly long night, not only were my legs cramped, but my hearing was almost gone. I was all but booking the appointment to get my tubes tied.

Get a Puppy

Dogs yap and cry and pee and poop and sleep whenever they feel like it, just like babies. And, like kids, they're born with their personalities, and to some degree, no matter how well you train them, they'll do what they want when they want. So having a dog will teach you *something*, at least, about responsibility and the cramp on your freedom that caring for another will cause. Bowie the wonder dog has certainly taught us how to contend with another's will.

Dogs also get sick. They teach you what to worry about and who to call. In the several months after we got Bowie the beagle, he'd had three ear infections and took more pills than Judy Garland used to. In order to manage all his maladies and their various prescriptions, I used charts and a complicated timer system. Yes, *charts* were necessary, on the off chance I forgot a pill or was struck by amnesia or my husband took over.

I try to think back to when my life wasn't dictated by canine pill schedules; when I didn't have dog poop under my

"I can honestly say there is nothing in the world I wouldn't do for my eight-year-old dog. States should require all potential parents to have a dog before having a child. Not a cat, a *dog*. People need training too."

—C.H., Fort Wayne, IN

fingernails; when I could leave the house for hours on end, make it a double feature at the movies, with no responsibilities tethering me back home; when I had time for manicures and facials and showers; and when, in lieu of my crusty sweats, I wore sexy back-baring shirts and three-inch heels. I was a different woman back then. It feels like decades ago, but it isn't even half a year.

That's right, our little internship in parenting is mere months old, and I can already say pet ownership is a double-edged sword. The advantages are that we now have some idea of what's in store for us when we do decide to embark on parenthood. The disadvantages are that we now have some idea of what's in store for us when we do decide to embark on parenthood.

Surrender

Bowie's favorite thing to do is to stand on my chest while I'm lying on the couch. He looks like the king of the mountain as he towers over me and stares into my eyes for a moment before the madness of his kissing begins. He licks my cheeks, my neck, my forehead, my nose, my teeth. The first few times he did this, I loved him as much as anyone I'd ever loved before. I laughed hysterically until a terrible wave of fear would overtake me. Almost as if his kissing could eventually consume me. Each time, I'd immediately sit up, unable to catch my breath.

I had a similar experience when he would come running toward me, tail wagging. Every time he came running, I spontaneously started to sweat. *He needs me*, I thought. I tried to duck behind the couch, but he busted me and ran to me with a tennis ball almost the size of his head in his mouth, expecting to play. My heart dropped. He wanted to play. That's all. He wanted company and I was hiding from him. The ball rolled out of his mouth and he chased it; then he tripped over his own feet and accidentally did a somersault. When he resurfaced, he quickly turned to search for me, while he wagged his tail to make sure I caught the excitement. "Get a load of me, Ma!" My heart ached with love for him, which made me feel even more guilty for hiding from him.

Bowie loves our sweaty T-shirts. They smell like us and he sucks on them at nighttime, like a binky. He loves us. Part of me is flattered, part of me is perplexed. *Already?* My husband can barely stand being at work during the day because he misses Bowie so much. And you can tell the puppy knows and loves my husband in kind.

I've been told I keep everyone at the slightest distance. I'm hesitant to let myself accept others' love. Maybe because I'd had one too many disappointing relationships or one too many times when my faith was tested and I took the leaps and fell flat on my face. Somewhere along the way, I decided to keep myself guarded, refusing to leap anymore. The less I cared, the less there was to lose. My husband was the exception to the rule. But now we had this little puppy trying to weasel his way into my heart, and all I could think of was how raising a dog is nothing *but* a

leap of faith. Last I heard dogs don't live forever, or, on av-
erage, much past fourteen. Inevitably, this will end. So part
of me wonders, why even invest in the first place?

I didn't think getting a dog would be this terrifying. I en-
visioned fetch. I didn't envision the emotions attached.

Bowie and I sat in the vet's office. He'd been scratching so
furiously I worried he would make himself bleed. Also,
patches of his fur were starting to fall out from odd
places—his snout and his underbelly. I was 99 percent certain, based on research I had done online, that he had
mange.

The vet's receptionist in the waiting room gawked at his
patchy fur and gave me looks as if I were putting out cigarettes on his face or something. She handed me a form to
fill out. I paused over the blank that asked for "primary
caregiver." Was that me? Oh, but did it have to be me? Now
when my friends would spring an impromptu Vegas trip on
me, I had to say, "I can't, it's not enough advance notice."
This wasn't how this was supposed to go, was it?

I looked around the clinic. They certainly could do a little public relations work or at least soundproof the walls:
howls of dogs echoed through the halls. I felt little Bowie
shaking against me. I hoped he couldn't feel me shaking
too. In the waiting room, big barking dogs whose paws
were about the size of Bowie were barely restrained by
their leashes and owners. There was a fat whippet that
looked like a pregnant supermodel.

A man came in with a slow-walking terrier of some sort.
The man had dark circles under his eyes, and just when I
thought I could relate, I realized his dog was not a puppy.
Far from it—his fur was grayed with age, his steps were

lethargic, and his eyes were at half-mast. And the owner didn't look much better. His eyes were puffy and red.

The powder blue walls were probably painted to pacify, only they didn't pacify Bowie or me as we waited and he whimpered. I held him and could feel his heart inside the barrel of his ribcage, banging like a drum.

"Rooster Clark?" the receptionist said. "That's us," the red-eyed man replied, barely able to restrain his tears.

"It'll just be another minute," she said. This seemed to make him cry harder. She gently pushed a box of Kleenex toward him.

He petted his dog and this seemed to soothe him—the owner, not the dog. The man looked at me holding little Bowie, then looked away. Bowie was watching them too, as if he knew what was happening. I held Bowie tighter. My heart beat so fast it could have exploded. Of course, my anxiety lay in the fact that someday we would be staring at these powder blue walls, trying to figure out how to stretch it just one more day, just a little more time, if not for him, then for us.

Bowie squirmed in my arms. I placed him on the floor, and he crawled right over to Rooster and licked the top of his head. Just when emotions were running high and things were getting too maudlin, Bowie lifted his leg and peed on the Wet Floor sign.

We were sent home after a diagnosis of mange and worms, armed with a pharmacy worth of pills, and the order to wash everything—all his bedding, toys, and towels.

Later, Bowie whimpered as he watched his bedding go around in the washing machine window. He seemed to be keeping an eye on Stephen's red shirt, Bowie's favorite, which he would suck on while he was asleep. He watched it go around and around, which made him dizzy, but he didn't give up. "My whole world's in there," his whimper said.

He knew I was watching him and came over to where I sat cross-legged on the floor and started to climb on my stomach, making me fall back. He stood on my chest and wagged his tail while he licked my face all over. I laughed, looked up at him, and I surrendered.

CHAPTER FOUR

Who's the Boss?

Ask your child what he wants for dinner only if he's buying.

—Fran Lebowitz

At a New Year's Day brunch, I got down on my knees to greet an acquaintance's four-year-old at her eye level. The little girl punched me in the mouth so hard I immediately tasted blood. What was more baffling was the mother's reaction: nothing to the child, but to me she said very sternly (as if talking to a child), "You really shouldn't talk down to kids."

Opinionoid:

Teaching children manners does not infringe on their individuality and freedom. Even apes have a social order with rules.

"Excuse me? And a happy 2005 to you too! Your child really shouldn't hit people!"

"She's a kid," the acquaintance said to me, without an ounce of apology in her voice.

"I don't understand," I said. "Is it too early to teach her not to punch people and learn some respect?"

Mommy Dearest went on to explain that "respect is a two-way street and you have to respect the child first."

"I don't really feel my *disrespect* warranted a fat lip," I told her. "And what's more, when is it ever going to be okay to hit anyone?"

Not surprisingly, she didn't have an answer for that.

Did this mother think her child was just going to out-grow this and magically turn into a good kid? And if she was letting her child rule the roost at four years old, what kind of hellion would that kid be at sixteen?

As I walked through the acquaintance's house, I couldn't help but notice that every surface was covered with stuffed animals, children's books, and DVDs. Children's artwork adorned every wall. The entire inside of their house looked like the outside of a refrigerator. Not one room was devoid of kid stuff. I felt dizzy, but I wasn't sure if it was from looking at all the brightly colored kid's para-phernalia or from being hit in the face. There was no sign that adults even lived there, and I couldn't get a sense of whom this couple was, other than parents to their chil-dren. Where had their identities gone and was this what I was destined to become?

It seems that in recent years, parents have given up the more traditional notions of parenting, swapping authority for permissiveness. And I've been watching my friends and acquaintances follow suit. Why are they letting this hap-pen? What are they so afraid of? Were the parents who

Factoid:

"From adversity, from limits, from no's, and from expectations, children develop greater depths of empathy, compassion, and understanding. Without these experiences, they develop a one-dimensional view of the world as the provider of what they want, when they want it. . . . Discipline is as much an act of love as cuddles and kisses. . . . It helps them learn how to fit in and accommodate the appropriate demands of life."

—Robert Shaw, MD, child and family
psychiatrist, and author of *The Epidemic*

raised them so awful? Were they all so horribly mistreated and deprived? I don't think so. So what's behind the overcompensation? Have parents forgotten that manners are necessary in the world and that children need to be taught that sometimes they have to do things they may not want to, like giving a cursory hello to mommy and daddy's friends or showing respect for elders? Children actually crave rules, and parents are the ones who must set them.

When I was a kid, if I had punched an adult, in front of my parents no less, I'd *still* be grounded.

As soon as the brat hit me, I considered walking right out of their goat-milk-gone-bad-smelling house. But instead, I decided to fill up on their expensive catered food. I have my priorities straight. I squeezed into a kiddie-sized Dora the Explorer chair in the living room and ate a quiche.

A few women were on the couch, the only adult-sized furniture in the room. One woman complained about the

lengthy application process to get little Breerly into
Waldorf's kindergarten. Another explained how hard it
was for them to sleep, since little McKenzie wasn't taking
to the family bed as well as their firstborn did. And another woman couldn't decide whether to plant baby
Bronwyn's placenta in the yard or to make placental soup.
I put down my quiche and tried my best to squeeze out of
the little chair.

As I was trying to wiggle my hips out of the tiny seat, the
women noticed me for the first time. "Do you have any
kids?" Placental Soup asked me. Not "Who are you," or
"What's your name."

"Oh, no kids yet," I said, my face flushing, mostly because of the energy I was exerting to get Dora the Explorer
off my ass.

"You will, don't worry," Family Bed said. Although I
think she meant it to sound encouraging, as if the only reason I might not yet have children is because of some sort of
physical difficulty, it sounded to me like a threat, as
though I'll one day soon be relegated to their couch, talking about whether I should make a roast out of my after-
birth. I nodded and excused myself, finally free from Dora's
embrace.

The men were huddled in the den watching one of the
college football bowl games on TV. I sat down next to my
husband, wishing I knew morse code and could tap out "I
weep for the future" on his thigh.

While the Toyota Capital One Outback Steakhouse
Carquest Doritos Bowl played, I wondered about our future: will we become permissive parents when it's our
turn?

———————

Friends have told me that the first time they held their child was one of the most profound moments of life. When I look into my baby's face, will the word "no" spontaneously leave my vocabulary? Will I allow my child to assault random party guests? Will I adopt one of the increasingly trendy parenting techniques I've been hearing so much about, like Attachment Parenting, Resources for Infant Educarers (RIE) technique, and principles of the Waldorf Schools, all of which focus on letting the child dictate what he wants, when he wants it? Many of the parents I know have insisted on labeling themselves with a "method" and taking their beliefs to almost cultish levels. So what's all the fuss about? I researched each of these methods to find out.

Attachment Parenting

My friend, Kay, and her husband, Roy, had a baby boy they named Maple Leaf. No, they weren't Canadian. They just really loved nature. This was news to me, since I once had to explain to Kay that hiking was just walking on an incline or decline. To which she responded, "Oh, so what's the point of doing it? Why don't we just get a drink instead?" My, how times changed.

Despite his unfortunate name, Maple is adorable and has huge hound-dog cheeks that any meddling aunt will someday want to pinch. He always smiles when I hold him, and I like to think it's love, even though I know it's just gas.

Roy and Kay are huge fans of the Attachment Parenting movement. So much so, that Kay has already tried to "sell me" on it twice: "Carrie, you and Stephen *must* become attachment parents when it's your turn. It's the best. I feel so at one with my baby!"

I smiled at her, as if I was waiting for a punch line. But she wasn't kidding. This was how she talked now. And she was so blasé about it, as if she were telling me there was a great new restaurant Stephen and I should try.

"Aww, I'm good," I said. "We're all set." What I wanted to say was that the whole thing sounded a little icky to me, like home births or yogurt you can drink.

Since when do people push their parenting techniques on you? Does she get a free toaster if I join her club? In order to understand my friend better, I read William Sears' philosophy of attachment parenting, the hallmarks of which are the five Bs: bonding, breastfeeding with a lengthy duration, babywearing, bedding with baby, and being responsive to your baby's cry. Attachment parenting encourages you to bond as much as possible with your child. Isn't that an innate desire? Extended breastfeeding is recommended, and the child can sleep in "the family bed" until he doesn't want to anymore. What if that's not until he's fifteen?

Kay and Roy have followed the attachment parenting guidelines to the letter: they never put the baby down. Baby Maple is constantly in their arms or in a sling attached to them. He sleeps between them in their bed at night. They're not putting him on a schedule because, as Kay said, "Maple tells us what he wants when he wants it." Kay and Roy refer to cribs as "baby cages."

Kay also stores her placenta and amniotic sac in her freezer. This isn't a tenet of attachment parenting; I just thought it was worth mentioning. Note to self: never have ice cream at their house.

When I questioned her about her devotion to attachment parenting, Kay said, "We don't want to hinder his development by putting our own expectations on him."

Oh gag me, I wanted to say. But instead, I asked gently, "What about promoting a healthy degree of separation?"

In the early morning hours, before Mom and Dad race in, doesn't baby learn to be content alone in his crib, which helps him learn self-control, focus, and self-comfort?

"The key is to let him know we value him and trust his instincts," Kay said, staring at Maple adoringly as he squirmed and grunted in his bunting.

"He's four months old. He's not seventeen! Aren't his needs pretty basic at this point?"

I wanted so badly to remind Kay of the kids and parents we used to hate for being so permissive, and now she was taking it to a whole new level! If she kept this up, how would darling Maple ever function in the real world?

Surely, there are other ways to bond with a child besides making him the boss and letting him dictate everything? And what happens to the spousal relationship? If you're all about your kids, aren't you literally putting your marriage and intimate relationship on the back burner? How will

"Look, I'm all for letting children develop unhindered. Let them paint pink skies and orange grass. Let them have imaginary friends and talk to stuffed animals. That's unhindered development. But refusing to establish boundaries—or making them paper-thin—is a poor way to help a child grow into a well-adjusted adult. If you want a kid to grow up normally, they need to get used to hearing 'no' once in a while. They're going to hear it when they're adults, so you might as well get them used to hearing it when they're kids."

—E.D., Indianapolis, IN

you ever have sex again? Or is Maple Leaf present for the conception of June Grass and Dog Wood? I'm nauseated just typing that.

And is all this attention and obsessive focus on kids really good for the kids themselves? How well adjusted is Maple going to be if he is the only first grader who still occasionally breastfeeds and sleeps with his parents?

It was at this point in the conversation that Kay then lifted her shirt and asked her infant son, "Do you want some milk, Maple Leaf?"

While she waited for him to answer, I watched in awe. If she was waiting for an answer from the baby, we might be waiting a long time, perhaps a few years. Maple merely gazed at her for a few moments, which sufficed, I suppose, as an "answer." Kay let the sucking begin. I saw this as a perfect time to give them some privacy.

I wondered if, in a few years, Kay's son would be hitting adults at holiday brunches and getting away with it because, after all, he was a kid and had to "follow his instincts?" Considering she'd just asked him for permission to feed him, it didn't seem so farfetched.

What does all this teach a child? That the world bends to them? That's not how the world works. Was she *trying* to raise a kid who wouldn't function well in society? This sure seemed to be the way to do it. Do you let him dictate the schedule and the rules of the house, dress him only in crunchy clothes, breastfeed him until second grade, and then send this poor kid out into the world?

When we were single, it was my job to be honest with Kay about boyfriends or career moves. But she was a mother now, and the rules had changed. This was her *child*. I couldn't say a thing. And I'd never been in the same situation, so who was I to tell her what not to do?

"If I raise a kid who doesn't function well out in the real world, whether it's in school or at a job or for general socialization, then it doesn't matter how attached I am to my kid, I didn't raise him well."

—S.D., Wheeling, WV

While Kay fed her baby, I scanned her bookshelves. There were at least thirty books on parenting—a buffet of different methods. On the one hand, I thought it was fantastic that my friend took parenting so seriously and had more than educated herself. On the other hand, I wondered: Whatever happened to plain old common-sense parenting? Our grandparents and parents—and centuries of parents before them—raised children without reading myriad books and committing to a child-rearing philosophy. So what happened to our generation that all of a sudden we felt we needed all this extra instruction and support? Were we products of our competitive generations? Were we trying to keep up with the Joneses? Or were more and more child psychologists and self-professed gurus trying to make a buck from this hyper-parenting trend by publishing books in hopes of starting a new craze?

Portions of each of these techniques seem counterintuitive to me. They suck the fun right out of parenting. What about following your instincts, figuring things out for yourself, and learning a few lessons along the way? Or are these techniques preying upon those who don't have or don't trust their parental instincts? Does that explain why so many people are worshipping Dr. Sears like he's L. Ron Hubbard?

I thought about Kay and Roy. Has recruiting others to their methods and ideals served to validate parents and their child-rearing choices? And why lecture others and try to convert them? I wondered if the fervor revealed insecurity—that's why they were uncomfortable with any deviations from the tenets.

While Kay took a shower, I spent some quality time with Maple. I baby danced with him, kissed his apple cheeks, and rocked him back and forth. As he slipped into a milk-drunk slumber, I turned my back on the bookshelves lined with tomes promising a healthy, well-adjusted child, and instead chose to savor my few precious moments with a sleeping newborn.

Resources for Infant Educarers

RIE is a parenting technique that was founded in 1978. I'm always dubious of parenting techniques that are younger than I am.

RIE is all about respecting the child. According to their website, following their instructions on how to become a good "educarer" and how to respect your infant results in an "authentic" child. (As opposed to what, an imaginary child? If I don't adhere to their guidance and training courses, I'll have a fake, run-of-the-mill kid?)

Many of the principles of RIE make a lot of sense, such as encouraging free play, allowing infants to work through their frustrations, and using passive, simple everyday objects as toys in order to raise more active kids. RIE believes you shouldn't interrupt a child, as this helps build his attention span. They appreciate and nurture curiosity in children and encourage parents to allow children to explore, thus discovering their own inherent abilities and building their self-confidence.

It all sounds good to me. But the RIE folks lose me when they tell parents—sorry, educarers—to "trust in baby's unique ability to show you the way," and "let your child develop naturally, according to his or her own rhythm." And then there's their recommendation to ask the newborn for permission before feeding, diapering, or lifting him, to show him you respect him—something I'd already seen Kay do. After asking Pumpkin if it's okay for mommy to lift him, you're then supposed to wait a beat for the infant's permission (which amounts to a moment of silence because *he's a freakin' newborn*), and then you pick him up. The RIE folks think this helps raise a confident infant and child, but I think this seems like a plan for raising a narcissistic brat who rules the roost. There has to be a better

"So this Alpha Mother comes up and says to her friend, 'You know, swings aren't RIE.' The friend, clearly not as strong a personality, mutters something about how she always uses the swing and that [her son] loves it. I said, 'Give me a break. Why is a swing not RIE?' 'Well,' Alpha Mother said, 'being in a swing is very passive and it is disrespectful to the child to put him in a place where he doesn't have the ability to get in and out by himself.' If you're into RIE that's great for you, but why come up to another mother, one who has made a decision for herself, and say *anything* to her about what is RIE or what is not? It's hard enough being a mother without someone else's inane questioning of her swing use."

—M.P., Santa Monica, CA

parenting method than one that insists you ask your new-born for permission to feed and dress him.

Waldorf Schools

Based on the philosophy of Rudolph Steiner, a scientist, artist, and philosopher, Waldorf schools are encouraged to "receive the children with reverence, educate them with love, send them forth in freedom." (Side note: Why are they called Waldorf? Are they named after Steiner's favorite salad or hotel?)

Waldorf schools structure their days differently than most elementary and middle schools. In the morning, children have a two-hour main lesson. For three or four weeks, they study a block from one of the core subjects (English, math, history, and science). Afternoons are devoted to games and sports, painting, handiwork, and gardening. Boys and girls learn crocheting and knitting, simple sewing, woodwork, and crafts. According to their website, the goal of "the Waldorf approach helps each student gain the inner and physical strength to flower into freethinking individuals. Artistic, cognitive, and practical lessons are all combined to nurture the strengths, potential and uniqueness of each child."

I love a lot of things about the Waldorf philosophy: I love that it values creativity and makes time for it (especially when more and more public and private schools are getting rid of recess and art programs). I think a child can learn as much about problem solving while building with blocks or working with a team in gym class as he or she would in a classroom. I think it's great that the philosophy fosters a love of learning. In my opinion, a thirst for knowledge is one of the best qualities children (and adults) can possess.

While knowing my child will be encouraged to express himself or herself through artistic projects or interpretive dance with no judgments, do I want that more than I want him to one day master pre-algebra? Not so much. The entire principle sounds a little like a hippie commune, except it costs 20K a year to send your kid there. And for 20K a year, I want my kid eventually to be prepared to take the SATs, not carve me a shoehorn.

Are these my choices? Hippie commune vs. rigorous college preparation starting in kindergarten where they do "drills and kills" and "teach to the test?" I don't want either for my nonexistent kids. Perhaps one of the biggest contributors to my pre-partum depression has been that I'm not prepared to make decisions like these and wonder if I ever will be. And what if I choose wrong? Will I end up raising a kid who lives with me until he's 50? Will he become a professional knitter because that's all he was trained to do?

"As a parent, you will make mistakes," my therapist told me. "You've got to understand there's no such thing as 'perfection' when it comes to child rearing."

I tried not to laugh. Was he telling a perfectionist to let go of her perfectionism? To relinquish her sense of control? That seemed like telling a fish not to swim or a fire not to burn! I nodded and waved him off, but deep down, I knew he was right. And this scared me even more.

The Self-Esteem Movement

During the interminable New Year's brunch, while hiding out in the den with the men watching sports, I over-

Pre-Partum Pointer: Beware of the Ever-Inflating Ego!

A study called "Egos Inflating Over Time," by Professor Jean Twenge (author of *Generation Me: Why Today's Young Americans Are More Confident, Assertive, Entitled—and More Miserable Than Ever Before*), examined the responses of over 16,000 college students from 1982 to 2006 and found that today's generation is the most self-centered in the history of America. Twenge and the study's co-authors trace the rise in narcissism back to the self-esteem movement in the 1980s and the increase of permissive parenting.

heard the hostess's husband narrating the exciting conclusion to his son's T-Ball season. "Oh," I said casually, joining the conversation late, "did Little M's team win?"

The husband looked at me as if I had just threatened to kill his whole family right then and there. "Carrie!" he whisper-yelled. "We don't use terms like that! We just coach the kids to have a good time."

"Are the two mutually exclusive?" I asked. "I mean, I had a lot of fun when I was playing kiddie soccer, even though we were trying to win." Our record was 0 and 12, I believe. I don't remember any of the losses vividly, but I do remember how much fun I had, running up and down the field, flailing my arms, and screaming "I'm open!" and then doing nothing with the ball once I had possession. No matter how many losses we amassed, we still showed up for every game and worked our little seven-year-old butts off.

———

Another parent recently told me that most of the kids in these scoreless games were still keeping score among themselves. The parents think they're making everybody (mostly themselves) feel good, but a certain amount of competitive spirit is not, in fact, a bad thing, and it makes it more fun for kids.

Obviously, the other extreme doesn't work either. No one wants to have one of those crazy Sports Dads or Stage Moms who yell at their kids from the sidelines or push them into an activity because they're frustrated by their own unfulfilled dreams. But competition is part of life, whether we like it or not. The world is a competitive place. Isn't it our responsibility, and the responsibility of schools, to prepare kids for the real world as best they can? Shouldn't children be taught how to handle competition?

You teach kids not by removing the competition, but by subjecting them to competition. This enables them to persist when they don't get the outcome they want. Better to encourage them after they lose than to spare them every form of competition entirely.

I was terrible at a great number of team sports over the years. My most notable failure was field hockey my freshman year of high school. I was truly awful and very skittish; I would actually run away from the ball. At the end of the season banquet, I was given the best-attitude certificate. I knew what this meant. It might as well have said: "You're terrible, but it's so nice that you refill the water bottles for us every game." But trying field hockey and failing miserably freed me up to pursue other, more solitary sports, like track and cross-country. I loved these sports and they got me recruited by colleges.

Sure, it sucked being the last one picked for gym class basketball teams, but it made me try harder. I practiced

> "Education researchers . . . decided that giving Johnny the C
> he earned would be bad for his self-esteem, and they decided
> he should get the A he didn't earn. As one observer puts it, 'If
> self-esteem is our goal, we're making our kids feel terrific
> about doing less and less.' "
>
> —Maureen Stout, Ph.D., *The Feel-Good*
> *Curriculum: The Dumbing Down of America's*
> *Kids in the Name of Self-Esteem*

basketball with my dad after dinner most nights, perfecting the now famous Friedman Free Throw, which included a great deal of prancing around while dribbling before shooting an air ball. I was never a star basketball player, but that wasn't the point: I was given a gift by not being chosen for the team, and that gift was playing basketball after dinner with my dad. It remains, to this day, one of my favorite pastimes with him.

In the sixth-grade student counsel election, I campaigned hard. I made hand-pressed buttons in our school colors that said Vote For Carrie. I got on my mom's fancy new Apple IIC computer that printed one whole dot matrix a minute and designed banners with witty campaign slogans such as "Don't Be Contrary, Vote for Carrie!" and "More Recess, More Fun: Vote Friedman."

With gems like that, I'm sure you're shocked that I lost. I didn't just lose, I was slaughtered. A fellow classmate who would go on to beat me in every single election for the next six years, won by a landslide. I was crushed, but I learned not to base my own self-worth on the opinions of others. And I'm proud to say that the loss didn't stop me from trying again and again and again.

My character and sense of self came from those moments just after being the last one picked for teams in gym class. Why? Because it required me to deal with those emotions and then pump myself back up. And that's a skill I use every day now. I learned how to cope with those feelings. When I got in the car that day and told my mom I had lost the election, she asked me, "Do you feel you did your best? Campaigned as hard as you could?"

"Yes," I blubbered through my tears.

"Then that's all you can control." That night, she made my favorite soup. Eventually, I felt armed with the tools necessary to rely on myself for my own self-worth. How cool was that?

My mom hadn't read any type of parenting advice book, but she just knew what to say. How? Was that an innate ability of my mother's? Was that part of her maternal instinct? How did we become so much less confident than our own parents in raising our children?

Now, in today's America, everyone's a winner. No one's a loser, but as the late George Carlin mocked, you're "the last winner."

In the den at the New Year's brunch, the built-in shelves are lined with kids' trophies, big and small. Some look like they might be chocolate on the inside. But the children are only four and six years old!

These days, kids get a blue ribbon just for showing up. So are competence and worthiness things of the past, now? Why are we trying so hard to soften the blows of losing? Why are we shielding kids from hard work? Determination? Perseverance? Aren't these qualities the building blocks for character?

School shouldn't be a therapy office. It should resemble a microcosm of the real world or, at the very least, prepare us for the real world: it's oriented toward results, competitive, and unfair sometimes, and you learn something new every day.

After the T-Ball talk at the New Year's brunch, Stephen didn't even bother with our usual party signal—he just handed me my coat. We quickly said our good-byes and as we walked to our car, he said under his breath, "I didn't think I'd make it a whole hour."

"That was only an hour?" I asked. It felt like days.

Once we were in the car, Stephen let out a huge sigh, then said, "I hereby declare that that NOT become a New Years' Day tradition, okay? Promise me we'll never have to do that again."

"Oh, I promise," I said. "I got punched in the face!"

"I got in trouble because I used the word 'no'," Stephen said.

"What? No?" I asked.

"Yes!" he said. "Apparently no is a banned word in their house! You're not allowed to say it. Mom and Dad think it's too negative."

"I thought that was the point of the word 'no.' What are they smoking?"

"I have no idea," Stephen said, "but there were so many other banned words of the four-letter variety I wanted to say when they told me that!"

What is going on here? Why are parents anesthetizing the world for kids? It's leading to a generation of shallow, easily disappointed kids with rotten personalities! (Sorry, overly ripe!)

I've put together a little glossary of other examples of child-proofed language (that actually, unfortunately, exist—see the box, opposite). You can probably overhear some of these at your local progressive school, where they call the teachers by their first names.

Glossary of Politically Correct Parenting

Traumatizing word: "No."
Apparent Problem: Negatively affects a child's development.
Alternative: "Stop."

Clearly debilitating statement: "I'm so proud of you, son!"
Apparent Problem: According to some child psychiatrists, phrasing it this way enforces the child's belief that they should seek your approval.
Alternative: "You must be proud of yourself, son."

Phrase that will scar them for life: "Good girl/good boy"
Apparent Problem: Sexist.
Crazy-Ass Alternative: "Congratulations!"

Horrific name for a children's pastime: Hide and seek.
Apparent Problem: Singling out the kid.
Alternative: "Be found if you want to be."

Flawed diagnosis of a child: Pyromaniac.
Apparent Problem: Labels can pigeonhole a kid.
Alternative: "A thermal enthusiast."

Violent and potentially fatal group activity: Dodgeball.
Apparent Problem: Encourages intolerance and bigotry.
Alternative: Sit in a circle in gym class, passing the talking stick around and airing out your feelings.

Torturous disciplinary action: Time-outs.
Apparent Problem: Alienating. (Isn't that the point of a time-out? "Go to your room and think about what you've done?")
Alternative: "You haven't done anything wrong because you're perfect, little pumpkin! Whatever impulse or desire you have is right even if it turns you into a serial killer later in life. Even then, I'll love you just the way you are!"

What I find most interesting and ironic about the self-esteem movement is that, according to most psychiatrists, these kids actually grow up to have *less* confidence, motivation, and self-esteem. These insecurities evolve from the feelings of abandonment kids feel when their parents aren't keeping them in check enough or preparing them adequately for the real world. The self-esteem movement potentially encourages kids to "act out" to try to find and define boundaries. So we're not doing the kids any favors.

And now we're seeing the results in the "millennial" generation, those born after 1980 who were raised being told by Mr. Rogers that they were "special," and receiving trophies just for participating. But it has been backfiring. According to a report by *60 Minutes* in November of 2007, the Millennials (called "narcissistic praise hounds" in the report) have weak work ethics and aren't prepared for the "cold realities of the workplace" once out of college, after lifetimes of being coddled. In fact, more than half of college seniors move back home after graduation. Companies are now hiring consultants solely to help them deal with this new generation of employees that "only takes yes for an answer." Bosses are finding they have to "motivate, train, and . . . nanny" this generation.

As we sped away from our New Year's hell, Stephen and I agreed this was not what we wanted our future to look like. And this unity made me happy—downright giddy—as we started a new year together on our own terms, far, far away from the nutty house where the word "no" was a no-no.

CHAPTER FIVE

The Insolence Hormone

*The problem with children is that you have to
put up with their parents.*
—CHARLES DELINT

Several years of observations of parents in their natural
habitats have led to my highly scientific discovery, the
Insolence Hormone. You're probably familiar with the
Insolence Hormone. Perhaps someone in your life suffers
from an Insolence Hormone imbalance, and therefore
you're well aware of the telltale symptoms of the chemical
change that turns normal women into momzillas.

The Insolence Hormone is most often released right after a woman gives birth. At that moment common courtesy flies the coop and in place of it is the "love me, love my
baby" syndrome.

Perhaps one of the most stunning examples of the
Insolence Hormone I ever saw was witnessing a formerly
kind, polite woman pitch a fit because store personnel
weren't allowing her adorable little one to play with the in-

credibly fragile glass ball ornaments at Bloomingdales. She wasn't always like this; she had once sneered at the obnoxious parents who brought their infants to fancy, adult, nighttime restaurants or R-rated movies and let them carry on.

Newly minted parents seldom recognize that their own off-putting behavior is terrible advertising for the club that they so desperately seem to want others to join.

Kids on a Plane

I was on my way to a friend's wedding on the East Coast and was flying solo because my husband's work schedule wouldn't allow him to join me. I knew I was in trouble as soon as I boarded the plane. Trying to find my seat, I kept checking the number printed on the ticket—20C. As I advanced down the airplane aisle and saw a mother with a child squirming all over her in the middle seat, my heart sank. I checked my ticket and the seat number obsessively. God, please let this be a mistake. I'd even take across the aisle. Anything. Just not next to the kid. But luck was not on my side. Sure enough, the child and his mother were *both* in seat 20 B—mom hadn't bought the kid his own seat. A man with a briefcase was crowded into the window seat, looking miserable. I think the airline rule is once your kid can walk, he must have his own seat. I could attest that the kid could walk because before we took off but as soon as I sat down, he was walking all over me.

Multiple Choice:

You're on a fully booked, cross-country plane flight in the aisle seat. Next to you, in the middle seat, is a mother with her too-big-not-to-have-his-own-seat toddler on her lap. Hence, said toddler is crawling all over you as if you're a jungle gym that happens to breathe, doing raspberries in your face. You just want to get caught up on your back issues of *In Style* magazine to learn how to steal Halle Berry's look, but this baby's all up in your business, stepping on your thighs and spitting his germs at you. Do you . . . ?

a. Kindly ask the parent to take care of her child.
b. Scream at the parent to control her child.
c. Respectfully ask the pilot to make a quick landing so you can disembark.

I chose (*a*) and learned that there are two types of people in this world: those who take things too personally, and those who don't take things personally enough. I was dealing with someone in the latter group. She smiled and shrugged a "what can you do?" shrug, which I misinterpreted as a "Me No Speako English" shrug since I couldn't imagine anyone who understood me merely shrugging. So I slowed down a little and spoke a bit louder—why do we always increase our volume when talking to non-English speakers?—and repeated in my nicest possible tone (too

"It's bad enough that they're allowed to ride in the main cabin and not sedated and stowed in baggage below. (I'm kidding.) But perhaps a separate section in the plane? Adults are in one half of the plane, and adults with children are in the other half? I'll fly whatever airline does this—I don't even care where they're going!"

—A.K., Ann Arbor, MI

nice, in retrospect), "Could you please keep him in your own personal space and off my lap?"

"I heard you the first time," she said. "But he's a kid. What can you do?"

After takeoff, mom breastfed the toddler in response to his incessant screaming, "I'm hungry! Give me food NOW!" She was letting it all hang out—the other, unused boob just hung there, dangerously close to the arm rest we both supposedly shared.

The poor man at the window seat glanced at me over the head of the mother and widened his eyes as if to say, "This is gonna be one long flight."

I would have offered the mother my aisle seat except that I'm claustrophobic, and I have a bladder the size of a bird's, so I get up every twenty minutes to use the lavatory.

I turned kitty-corner behind me and saw twin boys who were roughly 20B's age. The twins colored quietly in their seats while mom read a magazine. From where I sat, I could see she had brought along a bag of tricks: coloring books, snacks, videos. Double the children, none of the noise. I had to guess the difference was the parent.

Back in the crazy town that was 20B, the toddler slapped his mother's face repeatedly, as if it were a game. And his

---

"Don't set yourself up for failure when going on a trip: bring as many toys and books to occupy your kids as possible. Rent one of those DVD players they walk around the plane cabin offering for $5 and put on *Finding Nemo*. And if all else fails, there's always Benadryl, which I never leave home without!"

—C.N., pediatrician and parent, Houston, TX

mom just sat there, taking it. Every time he hit her and she didn't say a word, I winced. This boy was learning it was okay to hit. Just what our world needs. I wondered if I should say something. Maybe ask her why she was letting him hit her, but it wasn't my business. Sure, she was sort of making it my business, as the two of them were in the seat right next to me, and this child would likely grow up into a little monster who inhabited the same world as the rest of us. I've always feared for the future when I see parents allow this sort of behavior. I had to wonder—and not sound overly dramatic—if kids who brought guns to school were raised by parents like this. Maybe they were just slapped around by bullies in training like this because no one ever told them that wasn't okay.

I imagined that the word "no" was banned in 20B's house too. Instead, it was always "Yes, Butler," and "Okay, Butler," and "Mommy loves Butler." Of course, all of this left me with only one question: What the hell is up with kids names lately? Butler? As in, "the Butler did it?" Doesn't that make it too easy for bullies to come up with nicknames on the playground? He would be the butt, pun intended, of every joke. Whatever happened to strong, classic names like Sarah and John? Now, we've got dogs' names for kids: Rex, Grover, Dane, Muffy/Buffy/Duffy, Mitzy, Bubba, Clementine, Humphrey, Bogart, Chester, Daisy, Boo, Bishop, Ripley, Abner, Kosmo.

Stop the insanity! It seems, sometimes, like parents are all just trying to out-do each other; who can get the most ridiculous without being killed by their children once they're old enough to realize a mockery was made of their moniker. It's not funny, it's not cute, and parents are ensuring that their kids will hate them. Also, they're pre-determining their kids' career paths. "Paging Dr. Bubba

Quiz Yourself!

Band Name or Brand Name?
Prince Lionheart[1]
Parents of Invention[2]
Backyardigans[3]
Crayon Experience[4]
Barnyard Bandits[5]
Soldiers of Fortune[6]

_____

1. Brand. 2. Brand. 3. Brand. 4. Band. 5. Band. 6. Band.

Friedman" is never gonna happen (but "Whooza good dog, Bubba?" sounds just right). No law school will accept Bubba. Would *you* want your divorce or your heart surgery handled by someone named Mitzy or Boo? I didn't think so.

Despite my request at the beginning of the flight, Butler was still climbing all over me. I turned to the mom, and she gave me her signature, unapologetic "We're all in this together" shrug.

Yeah, we're not. One, I don't care if it takes a village to raise a child. This is a plane, not a village. Two, I don't have kids, and if I did, I would have done everything differently, starting with investing in an actual seat for him and the economy-size pack of Benadryl's extra drowsy formula instead of letting him crawl on strangers' laps. If her child crawls across the wrong person's lap and gets, say, a shove or a push, mom will learn the hard way that we're not all in this together. And three, I will tell my kid to behave. It won't be a discussion, request, or negotiation. It will be a command.

I realize it's no fun traveling with kids, especially with air pressure changes, restlessness, and tantrums. I always feel bad for those parents who are at their wit's end, trying so hard to calm baby or child, doing the baby dance up and down the aisle. I honestly want to give those parents a hug because they're clearly trying and doing their best. I understand you can't, ultimately, control your child. He's going to do what he's going to do. But you can come appropriately equipped, as evidenced by the twins' mom kitty-corner behind me, who was now keeping an eye on her napping twins while reading a romance novel.

In moments like these, don't you wish everyone had to pass some sort of thorough exam to obtain a license to raise kids? Isn't it odd that you need a license to manicure someone else's lawn or nails, but anyone can raise a child?

What if there were free and required YMCA classes for everyone expecting a child—much like driver's education—which not only taught the basics (how to hold, burp, and feed a baby) but also showed how to respond to different situations and emotions appropriately? This course could be taught by local child and family nurses, therapists, and physicians who could impart their wisdom, including the important fact that as children grow, they need to be held accountable for their actions and actually crave structure, boundaries, and routines.

What if you could revoke or suspend someone's parenting license for abuse and other dangerous and unacceptable behavior? They'd have to take courses, much like traffic school, to clear their record. And there could be refresher courses offered at eighteen through twenty-four months to remind the parents how to interact in a society that doesn't frankly care that they have a kid?

I put on my headphones and tried to drown out the sounds of the future wife beater in training. As an early birthday gift, my sister had given me a meditation CD and sweet-smelling incense sticks. "I can take a hint," I had told her.

The first half of the CD was waves that apparently had subliminal affirmations worked in, inaudible to the human ear, even though I spent a great deal of time and energy listening very hard for these affirmations and, thus, defeated the purpose of the relaxing sounding waves. The other half was silence save the occasional utterings of a Noo Yawk–accented mobster-reformed-sounding type. "*Reeelax yo moind.*" And he was calling himself Rama Das Lamana, but you knew it was really, like, Tony Craperelli or something. But who would take meditative advice from a guy named Tony Craperelli?

Tony Craperelli told me to live in the right now. I opened my eyes and looked at my "right now" and thought, "What if I didn't like the right now? What if the right now was full of stress and anxiety and what I fear will be a life sentence of insane children running across the laps of strangers on planes while I sip out of a flask that I explain to my kids is full of 'mommy's special happy juice'?" Tony Craperelli, in the next breath, tells me, "Just focus on the good *pots* of the present. Fuhgettabout the rest." I looked over at the child. He smashed his crackers then rubbed them all over his mom's shirt while she laughed.

I ripped off my headphones and frantically searched

through my carry-on for any sort of sedative—Benadryl, whatever. Not for the kid, but for me. Fortunately, the carry-on I brought on this particular flight was the same one I had used for my wedding almost two years prior. Digging through all the pockets, I found a fabulous hue of lipstick I'd thought was lost forever (it was like shopping in my own purse! Steal *this* look, Halle Berry!) and—thank *God* I'm so disorganized—a vial of Xanax my lovely doctor had prescribed for me a while ago for the days leading up to my wedding, just in case nerves got the best of me. They did not; hence, I had an almost full vial. I put one of the pills in my mouth and sucked on it as if it was a cough drop, relishing the bitter taste of it melting on my tongue. My concern that the pills had lost their efficacy was put to rest in ten short minutes, when the annoyances, while still there, suddenly felt padded, cushioned. I smiled a little and closed my eyes. Because of my very sensitive system, this tiny little pill quickly turned the airplane ride from hell into something of a pleasure cruise.

The mother in 20B got up from her seat exactly once to take Butler to the restroom. The businessman at the window seat, who had spent the majority of the flight pinned against the wall of the plane, rubbed his eyes and said to me, "At least now if the plane goes down, it's not *all* bad." I offered him a Xanax. A man clearly not typically prone to accepting drugs from strangers, he immediately and gratefully accepted.

The second half of the flight was softened by my mild sedative. I nodded off and jolted awake a dozen times while trying to sleep as I've never known where to put my head when sleeping on a plane. I did manage to have one very strange dream in which I was a toymaker who had created a line of what I called, in the dream, "Mental Health Dolls." There was Sally Sleeps a Lot, Bulimic Barbie, Stanley Starts Fires (matches not included), and Dissociative Deidre (seven distinct personalities; collect 'em all!).

The sugary juice drinks the mother had been feeding Butler the whole flight finally kicked in, and he spent his sugar high running up and down the aisle of the plane, until a stewardess told the mother to "try to control" her child. Mom pulled Butler onto her lap and, in the process, he smacked his head on the tray table. He did the countdown cry (everybody run; he's gonna blow!), and his face went from red to purple quicker than a mood ring before his cry erupted into full-on piercing screams.

Unfortunately, his tumble coincided with me—in my slightly drug-induced haze—thinking of Samuel L. Jackson's line from *Snakes on a Plane*. "I have had it with these mother-f——cking kids on this mother-f——cking plane!" I started to laugh. Hard. Mom pulled her little boy away from me.

"Stay away from her, Butler. She doesn't like kids."

I stopped laughing and suddenly felt bad. I turned to her.

"No, actually, I love kids. But just because your child is the center of YOUR universe doesn't mean he has to be the center of mine."

She rolled her eyes at me and buckled her son in with her. We landed shortly thereafter. I all but kissed the ground of the airport terminal, and I wasn't the least bit surprised later to see Butler climbing on the baggage conveyor belt and riding it while airport attendants chased him around and around. The mother looked mortified for the first time. I know I should have been glad, as she was in need of a wake-up call and wasn't doing the kid (or the world) any favors by inflicting him on others and not regulating his behavior. But seeing her face mostly made me very sad for her, as you got the feeling she had no idea how she'd gotten to this point and how she could make it better.

Of course, a few minutes later, she was yelling at the airport employees for chasing her kid because "He's just having fun! Let him have fun!" And just like that, as fast as I felt sad for her, the feeling was replaced with anger and disbelief. Some people are truly clueless and are too narcissistic even to realize it.

The Tsunami of Inappropriateness

I've been going through a phase where all I see are overentitled parents who make their kids extensions of their own narcissism. The parents need a time-out for taking their children to places they shouldn't be, like R-rated movies, adult restaurants, and adults-only parties.

These parents are everywhere, and there are so many of them that I'm starting to wonder if this is something that overtakes parents once they have kids, like a tsunami of inappropriateness.

For my twenty-eighth birthday, Kay showed up at my house, unannounced, thirty minutes before the scheduled time of the party I was single-handedly throwing. Worse, she had her screaming baby, Maple, in tow—the same screaming baby she had said, in so many words, she would *not* be bringing to my adult party.

She blew threw my front door with all her gear, gave no

explanation, and commanded me immediately to get her a mug of water, three quarters full, microwaved for a minute and thirty seconds. I quickly did it and then returned to my frantic last-minute party preparations, like arranging the food and getting dressed.

She unpacked and set up shop on my living room sofa and then, in typical RIE parenting fashion, asked baby Maple for permission to change his "diapee."

"And can you get Bowie out of here?" she called to me as I was getting ready. "Maple doesn't like dogs."

Excuse me? Whose home is it? If I had known she was bringing her child, I probably would have made different arrangements and penned the dog, since he loved babies. But I didn't know that and therefore was not about to chase my dog out of my own house. And how did she know Maple didn't like dogs? They never took Maple out of the house or let him touch anything that wasn't "made by the earth."

What happened to my friend? Had she always been this inconsiderate, but because there was only one of her I didn't notice or was she now using her child as an excuse for her crappy behavior?

And it's not just Kay. I've seen this sort of behavior a lot lately, like at adult restaurants when I'm trying to have an adult meal with other adults. Suddenly, you hear someone's precious babe carrying on, and Mom and Dad refuse to escort the child away from the table. Instead, they eat their meals, no doubt used to this sort of temper tantrum by now, oblivious or untroubled or both by the fact it's disrupting the meals of other paying patrons.

I recently read about Dan McCauley, the owner of a Chicago café, A Taste of Heaven, who posted a sign instructing that "children of all ages have to behave and use their indoor voices when coming to A Taste of Heaven." This led to many upset now former patrons but even more supporters. "Part of parenting is teaching kids they behave differently in a restaurant than they do on the play-ground," Mr. McCauley said in an interview. "If you send out energy that says I'm the only one that matters, it's go-ing to be a pretty chaotic world." Mr. McCauley is definitely my kind of guy.

People all over the country have begun online petitions trying to get their local restaurants divided into children and nonchildren sections, like smoking and nonsmoking.

Multiple Choice:

Million Dollar Baby is about to start. You have your pop-corn and your sweetie by your side. You're excited. The movie's up for lots of Oscars. As it starts, you notice a couple two rows ahead of you have their infant in a baby carrier. The kid starts to fuss and cry. Do you . . . ?

 a. Do the disembodied "shh."
 b. Tiptoe quietly over and ask them to leave.
 c. Leave the theater to find a cinema worker who can do *b*.
 d. Ignore it, even when the baby starts to wail and mom and dad refuse to miss a frame of the movie.

At one point or another, I've probably done all that I've mentioned. Why is it always at the quietest parts of the quietest films too? Nothing takes my husband and me out of Clint Eastwood's heartbreaking mercy-killing scene faster than someone's kid yelling "POOPIE HEAD!" at the screen. Parents assume their children will be fine, and then when they're not, most do nothing. Even those who *do* leave, you have to wonder what they were thinking in the first place—that the kid wouldn't wake up? That if the kid did wake up, would the kid respectfully play alone quietly in the dark of the baby carrier until the credits rolled? Why not be realistic and not ruin the times of other paying patrons, many of whom have planned ahead by securing and paying a babysitter so that they can escape the very screaming other peoples' kids are doing. Perhaps Poopie Head's parents should have reimbursed every other adult in the theater.

It's 100 percent likely that we don't find your kids as charming and adorable as you do. So don't inflict them on us.

Back at my party, guests started arriving and Bowie ran up to me with one of Maple's pacifiers in his mouth—inserted correct end out. It was quite a sight and my first instinct was to laugh, my second to scream. I chased him around until I retrieved it. Kay was livid and threw the pacifier into the trash.

When I stopped responding to her orders ("Throw this diaper away before your dog grabs it") and allowed myself to enjoy my own in-full-swing party, she got the hint and

---

Creative Concept: YojoMama.com

Are you out and about and trying to find a kid-friendly restaurant for lunch? Or are you trying to avoid kid-friendly places for lunch? A couple of clicks on your mobile phone will tell you where the nearest is!

finally left. Everyone at the party breathed a collective sigh of relief.

Don't bring your kid to an adult party when you're not sure if it's kid friendly or not. If the hosts don't invite your kid, they don't want or aren't equipped to have your kid there. If you don't want to get a babysitter, then stay home.

Kay left in a huff that night, and I was angry too. A few days later, she called and apologized for bringing Maple along with her. I told her it would have been fine had I been given some notice. She agreed. And I added, "And I would have insisted that you bring his playpen to keep Bowie away."

For days after, Bowie lovingly licked Maple's pacifier that I had fished out of the garbage and washed off. It was love at first bite.

TMI!

Whatever happened to simple birth announcements like:

> *Baby So and So was born to the So and So's on this magical date at this magical time, weighing X amount of pounds and measuring Y amount of inches! Everybody's happy and healthy! Here's a picture or three of our newest addition!*
>
> *Love, the So and So's*

When Reyna had her second baby, she sent out very expensive, fancy birth announcements with a precious pink ribbon at the top and the words "It's a Girl!" letterpressed

**Parent Peeve: Words and Phrases That Should
Never Appear in a Birth Announcement**

- Fluid
- Forceps
- Vaginal
- Episiotomy
- Mucus plug
- Birthing tub

into the thick stationery. When I opened the card, a few folded pages of single-spaced type fell out: a blow-by-blow account of the birth, from first contraction all the way to the baby's dramatic, gory entrance into the world seventy-two hours (and four newsletter-like pages) later. By the time I put the pages down, I was a sweaty mess and felt like I, myself, had given birth.

Unless we ask for it, could you spare us the details? Give us the pastel card with the photos of the miraculous end result and the Cliffs Notes version, and if we want to know more, we'll ask.

Reyna completed her birth packet with a photograph. And there are certain photographs that should be kept to oneself—no matter how close you are to your friends.

I was glad it was a beautiful experience for her, but I could sue for damages (nightmares and inability to keep my food down) for this, her head-on crowning shot with her toddler son, Cayden, looking on in what appears to be horror and disgust. Join the club, kid. I considered calling her up and unfriending her on the spot.

I'm sorry, but to this nonmother, this isn't a beautiful

portrait. This is torture by childbirth. My husband is still recovering from being shown a photo of his friend's wife pulling the child out of herself. "I saw so much more of her than I ever, EVER wanted. God, please make the image go away!" That shit sticks in your head whether you want it to or not. Now every time he sees her, he cringes a little.

While we're speaking about modesty, I don't want to see your ta-ta's either.

I am, of course, speaking about public breastfeeding. I understand that babies are on a schedule and have to eat often, including in public. But could mom use a little discretion and cover up? If I wanted to see another woman's boobs, I'd hang out in my gym's locker room more often or just become a lesbian. Seriously.

I realize I'm in the minority here. In a recent poll conducted by BabyCenter.com, 81 percent of the more than 57,000 people who voted think it's appropriate for a woman to breastfeed in a public place. In a related poll of breastfeeding moms, 60 percent were comfortable breastfeeding in public.

But come on, just because you've chosen to have a

Creative Concept: Hooter Hiders!®

In 2004, tired of modesty-compromising, unsightly, clinical nursing covers, Claire and Ronnie Ekelund created Bebe Au Lait and Hooter Hiders nursing covers. Made in beautiful, stylish fabrics, these nursing covers can be found in baby and maternity boutiques all over the world.

baby doesn't mean we have to look at your saucer-shaped areolas in the food court at our local mall, okay? I didn't buy this chicken Caesar wrap just to throw it back up.

Does the Insolence Hormone affect everyone? Is anyone immune? Will I someday be whipping out my ginormous milk-filled gazongas in the middle of an eatery? God, I hope not.

The Insolence Hormone doesn't only present itself at public events—it can also pop up during perfectly normal acts of common courtesy—like saying "thank you." I once sent a baby gift to an acquaintance, who promptly sent a note back explaining they had donated my gift to the Goodwill, as they're raising their little hippie in only organic clothes. (Last I checked, wasn't cotton organic?) A simple thanks would have sufficed.

Also, when I gave Reyna her baby daughter's gift in person, the words thank you seemed to have left Reyna's vocabulary. Reyna held up the outfit I purchased and said, "Oh, she's already outgrown it!" She put the outfit back into the box and handed it back to me, as if to say "Try again." (Buzzer sound.)

No, sorry! The correct answer was thank you. I knew Reyna could tell what store it was from, so why not return it and get the size or style she really wanted or save it to regift to someone else? But it was a gift. If I had to call her daughter Sailor-Jane for the rest of the time I knew her, the least she could do was accept a gift with grace.

"So many things can go wrong during births, whether the mother's in the hospital being kept under observation, being put under anesthesia, or walking around her apartment just preparing to deliver naturally. There is always the possibility of cord prolapse, cephalopelvic disproportion, breach or transverse presentations, fetal heart decelerations (strong indication of fetal distress), or placental abruption requiring emergency c-section. You never know what may happen during labor. It's completely out of your control. Not being as prepared as possible for the emergency situations is an awfully big risk to take with a child's life."

—L.L., OB-GYN, Winnetka, IL

Home Births

Home births and natural childbirths have recently come back into vogue, and while I can see the positive side of such choices, I have to wonder if the resurgence of the home-birthing movement is just another way narcissism rears its ugly head. I don't think it's just a coincidence that anyone I've ever known or heard of who has given birth at home also happens to have a photographer (or a videographer or both) present.

When Kay went into labor with Maple, first she called her professional photographer; then she called the midwife. This sort of exhibitionism is telling. *Look at me, look what I did.*

Kay raved about her home birth and offered even to show me the video. I declined before she finished asking the question. But then Reyna, a woman who, prior to this, had deemed herself "too posh to push," had a home water birth because she heard Cindy Crawford, her personal hero, had done it. And some of my relatives had given birth at home because they didn't have insurance. They too said it was a moving, beautiful experience. Maybe there was something I was missing?

I rented a documentary about home birthing, to see what all the fuss was about, and to make it more interesting for me, I grabbed a bottle of cabernet and turned it into a drinking game.

Every time a woman in the film described the home-birthing process in purely self-centered terms, I drank.

After nearly two hours of listening to gads of women wax poetic about "the empowering" experience of home birth and the way it was "giving the power back to the woman," I had finished the entire bottle of cabernet and was shouting at the screen: "Ish not about you, bishes!"

One woman mentioned "the gift you're giving your baby" but never said what that gift was, exactly. If there were differences between babies born at home and those born in hospitals under medical supervision, what, pray tell, were those differences? Because the documentary didn't say, it reaffirmed my belief that this wasn't about the babies at all, it was about the parents. The documentary failed to answer some other critical questions: why no fetal heart monitors and could they perform an emergency c-section right then and there if need be? These would have been valuable things to discuss, at the very least. So what if mom felt empowered pushing out her baby? That meant nothing if the baby was stillborn with the cord wrapped around its neck.

The documentary did explain that a lot of women who chose home births were doing so to prevent the unneces-

"This is not to say that there are never problems with hospital deliveries or that every home birth goes wrong. Not at all. But once you've seen a situation where you think, 'If only they'd been in the hospital . . .' it's really hard to get that out of your head."

—NICU nurse, Boston, MA

sary interventions that hospitals sometimes force on women, which made sense to me. But I didn't understand why women who chose home births wouldn't surround themselves with doctors just in case, God forbid, something didn't go according to their "birth plans."

Maternal narcissism aside, I was moved by this documentary. Each time a woman in the film gave birth, no matter if she was in a kiddie pool or in her bathtub, I burst into tears and got chills. (And not because of the searing screams of pain these women emitted.) Regardless of the motives of the mothers, the film showed life entering the world, and it was profound. I had to pause the DVD to grab tissues more than twice. It was the first time I realized that not only did I want to have a baby—but I wanted to experience childbirth.

I imagine that giving birth to a child naturally, in your own home, is one helluvan incredible feeling of accomplishment. But that said, I know things can go wrong. If I want to feel a sense of accomplishment, I'll run a marathon. There are lots of similarities between childbirth and running a marathon, actually: It takes tons of preparation, patience, and endurance. It's arduous, thrilling, painful, exhilarating. The biggest difference is, I'm the only person in a marathon. It doesn't affect anyone else. I just can't imagine endangering the life of another for my empowered feeling, no matter how profound.

Matthew McConaughey, when describing his son's birth to *OK!* magazine, said that he was very involved during his girlfriend's delivery. He was in between her legs, and when the pain got too great for her, he said, "We got tribal on it." Apparently "getting tribal on it" involved breaking out the bongo drums and turning up the volume on the Brazilian music. Somehow this was supposed to help his girlfriend push the baby out. After 60 hours of labor, they had a healthy baby via c-section. As far as birth plans go, the idea of having Matthew McConaughey between my legs—especially without his shirt on—seems like a great option. But if he were in my face, banging bongo drums while I'm trying to push something the size of a watermelon through a hole the size of a nickel, I would get tribal on *his* ass and rip his throat out in one grab.

Everyone has their own way of dealing with pain, and childbirth methods are deeply personal. What's important is that we have a choice. We're lucky we can decide how we want to give birth, whether it's at home naturally, on drugs, in a hospital, "getting tribal on it," or with a scheduled c-section. There's no shame in any of these. What works for my friend may not ultimately be my choice, and my choice wouldn't be right for my friend. While Reyna prefers sending out four-page birth announcements, I might stick with a simple postcard. To each her own. But when that choice affects others— whether it's the passenger next to you on a plane who doesn't want to be trampled by your child or the person blinded because they receive photos of your hoo-ha in the mail, perhaps we all need to make sure our Insolence Hormones are under control. Because as Dan McCauley of A Taste of Heaven said, we're not the only ones who matter.

CHAPTER SIX

Having My Cake and Eating It, Too

*It's not only children who grow. Parents do too.
As much as we watch to see what our children
do with their lives, they are watching us to see
what we do with ours. I can't tell my children to
reach for the sun. All I can do is reach for it,
myself.*

—JOYCE MAYNARD

My Barbies always had jobs. Mrs. Heart, of the Heart family (Barbie's brunette mommy friend in the drop-waisted pink dress with the hearts appliquéed on it) had boy and girl twin toddlers and, in my daily play fantasies anyway, a huge briefcase that she put in the trunk of the Heart family Cabriolet on her way to work. It was a tight fit.

Ken—or whatever Mr. Heart's name was—walked to work. He was the Al Gore of his generation.

In my fantasy play, Mrs. Heart dropped the kids off at day care or school and then went to work. What she did varied from day to day, subject to change based on my interests of

121

the moment. Usually, she was some sort of architect or interior decorator. She was a doctor during the week I wanted to be a doctor, which ended when I learned I'd have to study decades of biology and organic chemistry. At night, after she picked the kids up in the cute Cabriolet, she also picked up a pizza and Skipper, who was always hanging out at Barbie's house. (Side note: Who was Skipper, exactly? Barbie's kid sister or illegitimate daughter?) Skipper would babysit while Mr. and Mrs. Heart went to dinner and a movie, but the Hearts would get home in time to tuck the babies in at bedtime. I loved playing Heart Family because I felt Mrs. Heart had it all—at least in my limited opinion at the time: she loved her job and her husband and her twins, had a great car and, under that conservative drop-waisted dress, had a kick-ass body that she didn't even have to work out to maintain. As I said, fantasy play.

Never once, in any of my fantasies, was my Barbie jobless. She never wore sweats and hung out at the playground, except on weekends when she wasn't working. Of course, the fact that a working mom was raising me greatly influenced my play. My mother was a nurse and had trained and studied and obtained all the appropriate degrees (and then some). She loved what she did. She loved going to work, and she loved us. In elementary school, we were latchkey kids—we would ride home on the school bus together, and the three of us would let ourselves in and make ourselves snacks. Then at 5 P.M., Mom came home, and all four of us shared our days with each other. I learned by my mother's example that the best lesson you could teach children was that they should pursue their passions. Because my mom was fulfilled in her career and did what she loved, she was much more mentally present when she was physically present.

That was in the 1980s, and I wasn't in the minority—
many of my friends' mothers worked too. So why, then, in
the year 2009, were so many women leaving their careers
behind in favor of raising their families? What changed
since we were children—or even since we were in college—
that our peers who were, for the most part, raised with a
mind that they could get a job and develop a sense of inde-
pendence, were suddenly leaving the workplace in droves
to stay home and care for their children? It seems to go
against what all of us said we wanted back in college or in
the early days of our careers.

Some of the most intelligent women I know have decided to leave the workplace to stay home with their children. Kay used to be a full-time writer. Now she jokes that

"As a person who became a mother at age 39, I had an extremely full life before my daughter was born 16 months ago.
Still, I couldn't believe the comments I got from people when I
was (*oh, finally!*) pregnant. 'Are you staying home after she's
born?' Um . . . yeah, I went to f——cking law school to talk to
my kid about Massey v. Ferguson and read her Miranda warn-
ings every night before bed. There will be a new part of my
life, but it's a *part*. A huge, amazing, wonderful part, but still
just a part.

"I love my kid dearly, but I want her to be a confident person who knows that life doesn't revolve around offspring and
playdates and what she wants. I know by showing her how to
be an independent and interesting person, she will grow into
someone who will tell her own kids, 'No, I won't cancel my
golf game just because I feel guilty that I'm finally doing something without you hanging on my leg.'"

—M.W., Minneapolis, MN

all she's written in the last few years have been grocery lists. Reyna used to be a brilliant litigator. Lately, she'd only been mediating fights between her toddler, Cayden, and the family cat.

I've always appreciated their devotion to focusing on raising their children, but I have also sometimes wondered if it's hurting society as a whole that more and more of these highly educated women are choosing to stay home; that some of the most brilliant female minds of my generation are folding laundry and reciting the alphabet instead of pursuing the careers they were so good at, loved, and went into debt to train for.

Some stay-at-home mom friends of mine seem happy as can be, as if they have found their callings. But more stay-at-home friends than I'm comfortable counting have a kind of sadness in their eyes. They love raising their kids but speak with remorse about the fact they can go entire days without speaking more than three sentences to another adult. Some have quietly asked, "I went to college for *this*?"

This does nothing to reassure me that I should purchase a ticket and hop on the child-rearing roller coaster any time soon. Don't get me wrong—I think raising children is one of the most noble professions a person can have and one of the best things you can do for the world. Parenthood, I've gathered, is a full-time job with very few, if any, vacation days and shitty pay.

For many years, I was a babysitter and nanny for a wonderful family of five little boys. I loved these children. Each had their own unique personality and required different approaches: one loved to read his own bedtime story, another liked to make up a story as he went along, with me acting it out for him, our own kind of live-action, choose-your-own adventure story. A couple of them loved sports and were very physical, making it hard to keep up with them as they ran around the house. A couple of them were more sensitive and shy, following me from room to room like pups. One responded to time-outs for discipline, whereas another was unaffected by them. Instead, he responded when a privilege, like dessert or TV time, was taken away. One of the boys was a budding artist. When he was seven years old, he cut off a large chunk of his hair and sent it to me in an unmarked envelope with a drawing he'd made me. "At least it wasn't his ear!" my mom screamed at the time.

The boys were delightful, with the exception of a bad moment here or there, such as the time they invented a game called "Aim, Fire!" in which they'd direct their urine streams at me while taking their baths. You can bet your ass I gave them time-outs for that one. My memories of my time with the boys were wonderful. I ran into their father last year, and he told me the boys (most of whom are now young men) still remember when I'd "mail them to sleep." Just at the mention of it, my eyes welled up. I'd completely forgotten this nightly ritual I'd made up, and the boys, now in high school and college, still remembered it.

Mailing the kids to sleep went something like this: I'd "write a letter" on their stomachs (i.e., tickling them), and I'd put them in their envelopes (covering them with their comforters). Then I'd write the address on the envelope (more tickling), seal it with a kiss and a hug, and send them off to dreamland.

As much as I loved those kids, I was always happiest right after mailing them to sleep so I could sit down and take a breath. I was exhausted, and I wasn't even spending the whole day with them, just four or five hours at a time.

My arms ached from lifting them, and my head hurt from their screaming and talking over each other, each fighting to be heard. Then one of the babies would start to cry on the monitor, and I'd trudge back upstairs.

As I've watched most of my bright female friends leave the workplace to raise their kids, I've become worried: will I have to choose between my career and my future children? Are the two mutually exclusive? Lately, it sure looks that way.

I love children but I also love my job. I find my work incredibly fulfilling and know it would devastate me to give up such a large part of my self, my life. If I abandoned my own passions, I'd be miserable. If I were miserable, I wouldn't be the best mom I could be, and that would affect my child. The happiness of the primary caregiver is directly proportional to the happiness and well-being of the child.

> "I have a great 15-year-old daughter. I really love her. She's been a lot of fun and work. I also teach reading in public school, and I like that. I also study and compete in ballroom dance, I really like that. In fact, I do a lot of other things besides being a mom. I do them fairly well too. I am proud of it all. There is nothing worse than a woman with many purposes who stops having all but one purpose and does a pretty crummy job of it while exclaiming she has found her calling. Great, another woefully unskilled worker out there. As a teacher, I've seen some of their best work . . . and Chinese products are a threat?"
>
> —S.B., Plano, TX

That said, I've always wanted to be a hands-on parent. I've always wanted to play with my children and listen to them, and I don't want to miss a thing. They'll only be young once. But I also feel it'll be beneficial for them to see that mom is a happy person and has an identity independent of them. In addition to being the best mother I can possibly be, I still want to have a life of my own, with a career I actively pursue so that they will, I hope, learn by example that the goal of life is to discover and follow their own passions.

Which leads me to the question: *can a woman have it all?* Back when I was making my Barbie dolls be working mothers, I never assumed I *wouldn't* have a choice. I just assumed you could do it all. As an adult, though, I'm realizing that these choices aren't always crystal clear; they come with a trade-off.

Still, as I get closer to having kids, I'm no longer satisfied by the answer that "a woman *can* have it all, just not all at once." If that's true, then how did my mother and so many of my friends' mothers "do it all" almost thirty years ago, with virtually no outside help? Is it possible that we're moving backward instead of forward?

Yes, the feminist movement has given us more choices. But we still have sacrifices we have to make in order to follow any of those choices. And while one tends to think life is liberating with more choices, in a way it's the opposite— it can be paralyzing, at times. Is it possible that all the options and avenues now available to women are paralyzing my peers' ability to choose? Is it possible that when they look at their families and their careers and decide that if they can afford to stay home, they do, out of guilt? Or is the notion of choice proving to be a fallacy: a mother can work, but at what cost to her family?

"These were choices that didn't feel like choices at all . . . they came at the cost of our 'full human potential'. . . . What kind of life is it when you have to choose between becoming a mother and remaining yourself?"

—Judith Warner, *Perfect Madness: Motherhood in the Age of Anxiety*

Also, feminism didn't change biology: women still have the babies, nurse them, and need the recovery time. As much as we might like to, we can't just jump out of bed after a c-section or an episiotomy. The crucial career-building years are 25 to 44. So, too, are the crucial reproductive years for women.

Society doesn't exactly make it easy. In fact, it's so hard that some women feel they've been pushed out of the workforce, rather than opting out on their own. They work in all-or-nothing workplaces that aren't conducive to doing much else, let alone trying to balance the other full-time job of parenthood.

Factoid:

CareerBuilder.com's annual Mother's Day survey finds that:

- 43% of working moms are willing to take a pay cut if it allows them to spend more time with their children.
- 17% of surveyed mothers have missed three or more significant events in their child's life in the last year.
- 34% of mothers admit to spending less than three hours each day with their children.

> "We have to break down the actual barriers that prevent women from being full people in society, and not only end explicit discrimination, but build new institutions."
> —Betty Friedan

So how *does* a woman "have it all?" How does she have kids and a career? How is she supposed to make these choices? Perhaps workplaces could help out a bit. Perhaps major companies should provide child care on the premises so that parents can visit or play during their lunch break if they wish. Perhaps they could create *more* part-time positions, implement job-sharing positions, and allow telecommuting (saves gas too!). I realize these are difficult programs to put in practice, but wouldn't it be worth it, to give parents a chance to have it all?

"Guilt becomes your constant companion," Reyna once told me. "And it's guilt about any and every choice you make," she said. "You feel guilty for working, you feel guilty for not working, you feel guilty for not wanting to spend

> "I'd say I'm 'doing it all' except for the fact that most of my salary, from the job I love so much, goes to paying for child care. So in what way am I 'doing it all?' A nanny, another woman, puts my precious son to bed every night, and I miss him so much during the day that it hurts. Sometimes I wish I didn't love my job so much because then I could give it up without missing it. The guilt on all sides consumes me."
> —F.H., Orlando, FL

every waking minute with your kids. There's no winning with guilt. You're damned if you do, damned if you don't."

Kay told me that when filling out a medical form at a new doctor's office, one space on the form stumped her. "It said 'occupation,' Carrie, and for a second I almost wrote down milkmaid. Can I really call myself a writer now if I haven't written anything in over two years?" The minute she found out she was pregnant, Kay put the pen down and the nursery's valances up (but no crib, of course, because it's a baby cage). I told her she was a gifted writer and should give herself a break—after all, she was forming and raising a human being during those two critical years.

But deep down, I worried that would be me in a few years. I tried to tell myself I was more disciplined when it came to my career than Kay was. But was I? How could I know? I'd never held my own child in my arms before. I'd never had the sleepless nights that come with raising an infant. How could I know I wouldn't make the same choices, when confronted with work or my child? How could I know what I wanted? I couldn't. And that was the scariest part of all.

Ladies Who Lunch

I do most of my writing at coffee shops all over Los Angeles, which allows me to observe the growing numbers of a certain type of mother: she's a lady who lunches—all day long.

There's one woman in particular who I actually know. Or used to know. And for a while, I saw her quite often. Every morning at II A.M. she blew through the door with her cell phone against her ear as if it were another appendage, ordered her coffee with a flourish, and waited

"None of my friends work anymore. I went to a top-tier busi-ness school, and every woman I had been friends with there is now a stay-at-home mom. My friends and I now have two types of conversations on the rare occasions when we actually speak:

1. *The I-am-so-busy conversation:* "The nanny is watching Little X, but the nanny can't cook, and my usual caterer is booked, so now I have to cook for this weekend's cocktail party of the moms from my Mommy & Me group and their husbands, a group that I couldn't possi-bly include you and your husband in because you and I no longer have anything in common because you work (and don't have kids) and I don't work so that I can best manage the nanny's raising of my child."

2. *The I-am-checking-"call-nonmommy-friend"-off-my-to-do-list conversation:* This conversation usually happens on the rare occasions that Nanny has been furloughed, as my friends are craving adult interaction, and takes place in baby talk, because my friends are multitasking be-tween calling me and keeping Little X out of the bleach.

"I have time for neither of these conversations. If I am tak-ing time out of my workday, it is for something that I will derive some benefit from, either intellectually or socially. Instead, I am just angry and annoyed after these calls at the time wasted on the phone with people I used to enjoy and who used to be able to carry on a normal conversation."

—N.C., Chicago, IL

impatiently while proclaiming loudly, pointedly into the phone, something like, "Well, I'd be there on TIME if this BARISTA would hurry up and get me my LATTE!"

Almost ten years ago, she and I were in the same screen-writing class, when I had just moved out to Los Angeles. When she introduced herself to the whole class, she said she wanted to be a producer. We befriended one another instantly because we were the only women in a class with a chauvinist for a teacher. On our fifteen-minute class breaks, she and I would sneak out to the bar next door and have a drink. The second half of class produced writing as loopy as we were. Then one day, she stopped coming to class. She sent me an e-mail telling me she'd met the man of her dreams and his schedule was too busy to accommo-date her attending our writing workshop. This confused me, of course. Was she his girlfriend or his assistant? Why was she required to go on all his business trips with him? Or was she electing to go on all his trips with him? The lat-ter seemed more likely. And after that, she seemed almost relieved that she didn't have to pursue that bothersome career-of-her-own thingie she had initially wanted. She was taken care of, and you got the feeling it wasn't a mo-ment too soon. We kept in sporadic e-touch for another few months, and then fell out of contact before she mar-ried him in a tiny ceremony on an even tinier island in the Caribbean. I read about it in the *New York Times*. In the article, they described her as an "aspiring producer and socialite."

Of course, at the coffee shop she didn't recognize me, and I never approached her—just watched her from my perch. Her once pretty features were frozen in place by Botox, and her eyebrows were plucked into a perpetual look of surprise.

She presented herself as a terribly busy woman, even though she had "people" who handled everything in every area of her life. I overheard her managing her staff on her phone each morning. When she wasn't talking to the nanny, the concierge, or the personal assistant, she was managing all the different *elective* dramas and commitments she had gotten herself into: fund-raisers for Harmony's no doubt already ridiculously expensive private school; tennis lessons for Rhythm, the 18-month-old; and feline therapy for Fluffers who seemed so depressed lately.

When her latte was ready, she grabbed it with an aggravated, "finally!" and walked out to her waiting SUV with its "My Child Is Student of the Month at The Beverly School" sticker on the back.

"You're overthinking parenthood," Reyna said to me when I confessed my fears during one of our visits. As she said this, two different nannies scurried in the background to attend to her baby's crying and her toddler's meltdown. Reyna didn't even flinch, didn't even blink. These people were basically doing all the heavy lifting. They were the ones getting up in the middle of the night and taking her

---

Parent Peeve

If you have round-the-clock help and you don't work, you can't complain about how busy you are. We know you've got a small team of nannies who live in your house, and the whole reason you got them is so you'd have more than enough time to nap and read and make calls. We know one of them is soothing your baby to sleep at this very moment as you get your second massage this week. It's all good, just don't complain about how busy you are. You know who's truly busy? The single mother of three who's working full-time and still can't afford an eighth of the help you have.

darling babes to Mommy & Me and doctors appointments and dance class. Of course Reyna thought I was overthinking parenthood—because in her mind, there was nothing to do!

Many women have sought out this lifestyle. To me, this is the threat of what can happen to a once perfectly interesting woman out here. This is my worst fear.

Once, one of my husband's friends asked me, "What do you do all day long? Yoga? Manicures? I swear, you and my wife have the life."

I didn't know which was more upsetting—being put in the same sentence (and therefore category) as his wife who did, as far as I could tell, lunch all day long or knowing he was my husband's friend, which prevented me from smashing his face into his balls.

Yes, I do technically stay at home. However, I'm working ten hours a day—it just happens to be out of my den.

Every time I watched my former classmate drive away from the coffee shop, I felt vaguely nauseated, and I mentioned this to my therapist.

"The woman makes you nauseated?" he asked me in my session the next day. "Why?"

There were so many reasons. I left out all the superficial ones, like the fact her face was pulled so tight it looked like a trampoline. Or that she was a clichéd trophy wife now who existed to manage her staff of helpers and keep herself occupied with projects like supervising the redecorating or rebuilding of the house. I boiled it down to this: "She once had big dreams for herself, and now, she doesn't seem to. It makes me equate parenthood with a total loss of goals and ambition. I see bringing another life into this world as an end to my own life as I know it. I know it's wrong, but I do."

I told him all about how Kay hadn't written a single nongrocery-listed word since her child was born. And she had given up her den to be a nursery, so she no longer had a room of her own in which to write. I told him about how Reyna, who graduated summa cum laude from Princeton and was at the top of her class at law school, was now memorizing songs from her son's pre-school class.

"So what?" my therapist said. "Those were their choices. You don't have to make their decisions. No one's asking you to live their lives."

"But," I said, "if you had asked Reyna and Kay a few years ago if they'd want to someday become full-time mothers, they'd have said no, vehemently! So who's to say that won't happen to me?"

I secretly feared I'd be the same way as my friends: so in love with my child and the new job of parenthood that I'd completely forget about my career, the one thing that had been with me all my life, through good times and especially bad times. I worried my passion for my career would just evaporate when the second job, which involved a "bundle of joy," came into the picture. I worried I would quietly fade into a routine with my children and be in some doctor's office two years from now drawing a blank on the career question like Kay. Or I worried I would try to fool myself and others into thinking I was terribly busy like the ladies who lunched.

"Nothing like that can happen without your permission," my therapist said. "The fact that you're aware of it right now—and actualizing it as a thought and concern—is a sign that you'll be even more aware of it whenever the time comes for you to start a family. Once you have a child, you'll make a choice that works for you."

And while this made me feel the slightest bit better, I

knew that by having children I'd be entering an unknown world full of all new emotions, and deep down, I was most afraid of how much I'd feel and what those feelings for this new human being would turn my life into.

The Myth of Having It All

Later that week, at the hair salon, I flipped through the kind of magazine I'd never buy myself but relished looking at when I was at the hairdresser. I stopped on a page that described a celebrity mother with a young child, a thriving career, and a perfect body. "She's truly doing it all!" the article proclaimed.

Really?

Nowhere did it mention the staff of people who were no doubt helping her do it all: the twenty-four-hour live-in nannies, the maids, the chef, the personal clothes shopper, the personal grocery shopper, the trainer, the publicist, the agents, the makeup people, and the live-in stylist who blew out her hair every morning.

And yet, I continued reading, falling victim once again to the glossy magazine portrayal of parenthood. Suddenly, I was mesmerized, subconsciously hoping to glean some tips on how to be more like this star who makes $10 million per movie. "Use your baby as a weight and lift him! Three sets of 40 reps a day, and you're on your way to tighter arms!" (By the way, who cleaned up the baby vomit after the 40 reps?) I read with the hope that she was, in fact, able to do it all. Because if she couldn't, with all that assistance, what was it going to be like for the rest of us, who couldn't afford or didn't want all that help?

I snapped out of my reverie when the hair stylist asked what I was reading.

"Oh, you know," I said. "Trash and lies."

While the stylist washed my hair, I shut my eyes against the images in the magazine and tried to recall the uncomplicated joy and blissful sense of control I felt when playing with Barbie, Ken, and Mrs. Heart all those years ago when the dolls took the risks and lived the lives I one day wanted.

CHAPTER SEVEN

Hyper-Parenting

Until recently, the essential tasks of parenting were seen as nurturing and socializing children. Today, however, this simple mandate seems criminally neglectful. Now, parenting requires constant vigilance, unflagging attention to every detail of our children's lives, and ever-present monitoring of their every activity.

—Katie Allison Granju

Kay's little boy, Maple, was seated in a grocery cart wearing what appeared to be a hazmat suit. I thought of the line in *Annie Hall* when Woody Allen asked his friend, "Max, are we driving through Plutonium?" Upon further examination, Maple seemed to be shrouded in a kind of shopping-cart seat cover. Why was this necessary? And how did the millions of us who grew up sitting in shopping carts without the crazy germ insulation somehow manage to survive intact? Were parents today being made to think these

139

items were required, by the corporations who—imagine this—wanted to sell these things?

Over the years, I have watched as more than a few of my friends have been kidnapped and swept away to some crazy planet, Planet OverParent. And with each new wave of phobias and worries, their actions have gotten wackier and wackier.

Overprotection

"I think she has a temperature. I'm going to take her temperature again. She feels warm." My friend Reyna grabbed my hand and pressed it against her daughter's forehead. "Doesn't Sailor-Jane feel warm? It's probably rheumatic fever. I should call the doctor. Oh, it's tummy time. I'll call her doctor after. She looks gassy. That's the face she makes when she's gassy. Here's a gas relief drop just in case. Are your little toothies hurting? She's teething. Here's some liquid baby Tylenol, poor sweet Sailor. Carrie, can you grab me some disinfectant for the thermometer?"

Not even four years ago, Reyna was doing bodyshots off a total stranger. Now she was orbiting around her second

---

"Should we don scrubs every time we leave the house? Nope. If we set that as our goal, a vulnerable infant's needs would be unlimited; someone somewhere has been hurt by everything, even things that under almost every condition are considered safe."

—Alvin Rosenfeld, MD, author of *The Over-Scheduled Child: Avoiding the Hyper-Parenting Trap* baby like a mobile, even though the baby had a mobile doing that already. She had given her child three drugs in the last three minutes.

When a worker from the phone company came inside her house to fix a phone jack, Reyna briskly left the room and reappeared after he'd gone, holding baby Sailor, who was now dressed in a different outfit. "Every person brings different germs into the house," she explained to me. "Every one has their own aura of germs that cling to your clothes."

I imagined all of us looking like Pigpen from the Peanuts cartoons, with our "auras of germs" swarming around us.

Who was this person? What had happened to my friend? This was her second child! You'd think, after her first child, she'd have realized, "Wow, he survived everything, including going outdoors and being exposed to other peoples' auras of germs, so maybe I should loosen up a little with this second baby?" But it seemed to be the opposite. She treated her baby girl as if she would shatter into a million pieces at any moment. I've always heard that nervous parents raised nervous kids because the babies could pick up on the energy. And then I witnessed it: every time Reyna tensed while holding the baby, Sailor started to cry. And when Reyna wasn't freaking the kid out, she was waking her up.

"A schedule is very important for an infant," Reyna told me as we stood outside Sailor's nautically themed nursery. I nodded, I had heard this before. Something about sleep training. Just as I thought I understood, Reyna opened the door to the nursery, swooped in, lifted Sailor out of her crib, and jolted the baby awake.

"Her nap can only be thirty minutes long, otherwise she'll never go down at night." The baby clearly didn't agree and wailed her head off.

I realize that I haven't had kids and haven't studied sleep training, but was it wise to wake a sleeping baby, and so abruptly? Were all these methods and programs and germ precautions actually weakening both the immunity and the tolerance of the child? Instead of raising a resilient, adaptable child, was my friend raising a future nervous wreck?

For all of Reyna's hang-ups, Kay wasn't much better. Kay and Roy forbid plastic in their house. "With the exception of newer plastics made from corn," Kay told me as we walked through the grocery store with Maple in the cart in his hazmat suit. "Even 'safe' plastics seem like a bad idea when they can be avoided. And they're not biodegradable."

What about toys? I asked her. Aren't a lot of toys made of some sort of plastic?

She told me about a new line of wood and natural fiber toys that were "less formed to encourage imagination." I had to look away for fear of rolling my eyes. I wondered: What did they think would happen if little Maple touched a G.I. Joe figurine? Would his hands melt away, as if covered in acid? What about when Maple went to his friends' houses? They couldn't regulate what he played with there. Would the boy live in a bubble? Of course, it would have to be a nonplastic bubble. Maybe it should be glass. I wanted to remind Kay that shielding kids from all these materials—while I knew the intent was good—was a little fruitless, considering he'd inevitably encounter them at some point in the future, anyway, when he was out in the real world.

I wonder if Kay has taken the green movement a titch too far. Of course, her conservationism is great. We all need to be more conscientious of our carbon footprint and energy use. But when you're sewing your son's clothes out of old washcloths and blankets, enough is enough.

I like to think of the green movement as a color spectrum. If Al Gore is a strong kelly green and Ed Begley, Jr., who lives in an all green house and rides on a stationary bike in order to power his toaster, is a deep hunter green, I'd say I'm a chartreuse: I only drive when it's too far to walk, I own a fuel-efficient car, and I thought *The Inconvenient Truth* was a very important movie.

In stark contrast to my chartreuse, Kay is a swampy, very dark olive green. She is so far along on the color spectrum and such a dark shade of green, it's almost another color—and movement—entirely. If you took away the fact that she has a lovely three-bedroom apartment in a nice neighborhood in Los Angeles, Kay, Roy, and Maple would be living in the woods. She only permits her family to eat food "from the earth." She and Roy keep a garden off their balcony where they grow most of their food.

Once, when their plants were going out of season, they called me and asked if I wanted to come over and do some composting with them. I've never had any idea what that was, but the word reminded me of shoveling horse manure, my punishment at camp one summer for trying to hitchhike home. I politely declined.

Kay and Roy said they got into this because they wanted to raise their son "pesticide free" (who doesn't?) and to them, that meant growing their own food in ecologically responsible ways. Okay. But eventually, the kid will probably get his hands on a juicy hamburger, and he'll love it. He'll eventually wear polyester, whether it's because he has a summer job at the multiplex movie theater or because he likes it. And all that water they use to wash his cloth diapers is a colossal waste of water and energy. Eventually, Maple will go to school and someone will offer to trade him some cookies from their lunch for something

Budding Brainchild: Combat Pollution by Starting with Yourself!

In just twenty minutes at my local, ritzy organic grocery store, I overheard two different mothers (with children present) screaming at store workers. One commanded the produce guy to clean her carrots; another screamed at the deli clerk because he had "promised there'd be meatless lasagna today!" There was something ironic about degrading and humiliating another human being while packing everything-free milk and paper towels into the back of the hybrid SUV. This demeaning behavior was toxic in itself. If they were so bent on saving the world, why didn't they start with their own behavior? (And maybe stop injecting botulism into their faces.)

in Maple's lunch. (Although, what they would trade it for I have no idea. Fennel?) Maple will discover sugar and he will love it. Why not teach him moderation with such things *now*, while he still lives under your roof, instead of having a college kid with Type 2 Diabetes?

When I was little, there was one kid like Maple in my class. Her mother sent her to school with the weirdest shit to eat—we're talking nuts and twigs here. Everyone felt sorry for the girl, and she was embarrassed and probably wished she had juice boxes and sandwiches like the rest of us. Her mother was a hippie and playdates at her house were always pretty miserable because the mom would test out some sugar-free bran cookies on us (that tasted fresh out of a wood chipper), and I'd be up all night trying to digest them. And the mom was anti-everything—anti-germ, antibacterial, anti-meat, anti-dairy, anti-taste.

At the time, this girl and her mother were the only people in our school who were like this, and it was considered strange. Now, twenty-five years later, this sort of behavior is far more prevalent. In fact, it may be the new norm. My question is, why? Why this insidious, mass hysteria about toxins and disease? Just watching a half hour of TV now means we're bombarded with drug commercials for ailments we probably don't have but convince ourselves we do. Then we ask our doctor for a prescription, as the ad suggests, and barely listen to the fine-print announcer telling us that "side effects may include stroke or even death." Gee. Makes you want to rethink how bothersome those restless legs are, no?

The media with its "if it bleeds it leads" philosophy, the government with its color-coded terror level charts, and corporations with their desire to scare us into buying stuff we need to "keep us protected" have created this hysterical culture of fear, and we're passing that along to our children.

I realize I'm a tad numb to fear and hysteria, as I was raised by my mother, who makes sure to tell us about the latest risks of living every chance she gets. The other day I got the following voice mail from her:

"Throw out all your flip-flops immediately! They only absorb germs! And you've got to get checked for heart disease! It can go undetected and then one day you'll just drop dead! Call me! It's mom."

I called her back. "You know what else causes heart disease? Your voicemails. Instead of leaving me these scary messages, why don't you just routinely jump out of a closet when I least expect it wearing a mask and brandishing a butcher knife?"

> "Too often we give children answers to remember rather than problems to solve."
>
> —Roger Lewin

Overprogramming

We were at some friends' house, where we watched their eight-year-old son, Jeremiah, as he played the violin. There he was, performing a freakin' concerto in their living room, and while it was wildly impressive, something about it made me uncomfortable. Once we were in the car, Stephen was able to put it into words for me. "I've never seen a child who looked suicidal before, but I guess there's a first time for everything," he said.

This was the same kid who said a few years ago that he was feeling "stressed out" (his words) about his upcoming kindergarten entrance exam. A few years before that, Jeremiah's parents were trying to weigh the pros and cons of certain "college preparatory pre-schools."

In my pre-school days, I was singing songs about the people in my neighborhood. Shouldn't pre-school be fun and at least foster a love of learning? Wasn't it counterproductive if my kid could recite Shakespeare at six years old, but despised school?

Before we'd left the friends' house, as I was passing through the kitchen, I saw a dry erase calendar on their fridge that had so much writing on it I thought it was a collage. Jeremiah had quite the social calendar for an eight-year-old. At least two days a week had "J playdate with" different names written on.

Every moment of little Jeremiah's life was scheduled, including play. Playtimes and playdates were on the calendar weeks in advance. And on other days, it said things like "J Karate" and "J math tutor." Where was the time to be spontaneous? Or was that scheduled too? As the late George Carlin once said, "When's a kid ever get to sit in the yard and play with a stick anymore?" Most children nowadays have never had the opportunity to be bored. If they aren't being shuttled from one activity to another, then they are in front of a TV or video game. Gone are the days of daydreaming. Every single one of my passions in my adulthood—writing, decorating, designing, crafting, drawing—was borne out of being bored when I was a child, or, more accurately, during unstructured playtime.

No wonder Jeremiah looked so exhausted and depressed. Because at eight years old he already had a longer, more impressive resume than I had when I was applying to colleges. I understood trying to become as well-rounded as possible in order to get into the college of your choice—but starting that at eight years old or earlier? What would be accomplished by having more extracurricular activities and fewer free moments in the day? Why had so many parents become such hovering presences, starting with playing Mozart for the baby in the womb? If there was no time to play or reflect, then how could a child ever be comfortable alone? It has been suggested that kids learn best through simple playtime, as it teaches problem solving, social development, and creativity, but now children are surrounded by continuous, frenetic activity. And we wonder why more and more kids have been diagnosed with ADD?

Why wasn't young Jeremiah playing with Matchbox cars or climbing trees? He was at the age to do those things. He'd only get one childhood, and here he was, spending it thrust into the adult world, playing adult concertos.

> "Play is to early childhood as gas is to a car."
> —Kathy Hirsh-Pasek and Roberta Michnick Golinkoff,
> authors of *Einstein Never Used Flashcards*

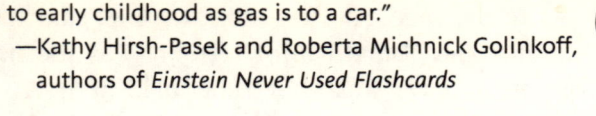

When did all this overprogramming start? Two year olds are encouraged to be trilingual, first graders are either medicated or sent to therapy or both if they can't settle down immediately after recess. Are parents today over-compensating? And why? Are they trying to keep up with the Joneses? Is it a subconscious way to undo what they feel their own parents have done wrong? Are they jumping into having kids too soon? Are they using their kids to act out the competitiveness and drive they might have directed otherwise toward a career? Are they allowing themselves to get caught up in this dog-eat-dog society where one person's success is another's failure? Isn't this a prescription for not only overstressed kids but also their parents?

Creative Concept: Childhood Is Calling™

Kellogg's Rice Krispies cereal has released a report called *Childhood Is Calling: Celebrating Kids Just Being Kids* that offers expert advice for families to find those ever-important simple moments of joy and connection. "The report helps parents take comfort in knowing that every single moment doesn't have to be a teaching moment and that some of the most valuable lessons that children learn are through self-directed, free play."

I couldn't necessarily fault Jeremiah's parents because I haven't been in their position yet. I imagine it's very hard to sit back and watch your child's classmates learning their third language or their latest sport without feeling like you should be doing the same thing. After all, one day—even if it's ten years from now—your child will be applying to college at the same time that kid will be.

I can find competition in just about anything. When jogging at my local track, I'll spot someone half a lap ahead of me and set my goal to catch up and pass that jogger by the end of my run. I won't let myself stop running until I've achieved this goal. When my sister and I were younger, we shared a bathroom between our bedrooms. In the mornings, when we'd both be groggy, facing the mirror and brushing our teeth, we'd suddenly catch each other's glance in the mirror and turn the teeth brushing into a race. Speed wasn't the only factor. Form was key. We'd pretend-narrate with golf-announcer-type voices about who won, who spit first, who displayed the best technique with their brush strokes.

So knowing I can make a competition out of anything, I'm a bit worried I'll get caught up in all of this "my kid should have gotten into the pre-school/private school/college/ballet class that your kid got into." On the surface I don't want that, but I worry the pull will be too strong and I'll become so involved in the rat race that I start to live vicariously through my kids. I know myself: I'm an extremist. I can't do anything less than 100 percent. What if I start to feel lonely, empty, and lost without my child defining my life? What if I get so caught up in the daily dramas of my child's life that they become the dramas in *my* life? Is this what my friends are going through? What's making them into such hyper-parenting nuts?

"You have to vigilantly hold on to your own sense of self," my therapist told me. "Too often, parents—mothers especially, as they are more often than not the primary caregivers—reduce their interests to one: their child. They give them all their focus, which is too much pressure on a child."

Even if I white knuckled my identity, I knew it would be hard not to get caught up in the overparenting craze. Like peer pressure for adults, the "everybody's doing it" element of hyper-parenting would make it harder to resist. Even though I snickered at it now, was it possible that I'd suddenly want to become an ecologically responsible farmer and only let my kid eat food from the earth, or buy grocery cart covers in bulk, or attach a thermometer to him that takes his temperature every thirty minutes to be sure he's okay? Maybe I would decide my child was gifted and would devote my entire life to getting him into Yale and teaching him to play the cello as well as Yo-Yo Ma.

Deep down, I was starting to suspect that when my therapist told me to relinquish control, this is what he meant. Either my kid would want to play the cello or he wouldn't, and nothing good would come of forcing it on him.

How could I be a good parent when I couldn't stand the thought of relinquishing control?

"Once you have a little offspring, if I ask you how you are, I expect to hear a sentence about YOU. Not the spawn. YOU."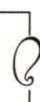

—A.M., San Francisco, CA

CHAPTER EIGHT

Fear

Most of us become parents long before we have stopped being children.
> —MIGNON MCLAUGHLIN

A girlfriend and I made a promise when we were twenty-four: we would not start having kids until we were thirty or older. This, we decided, would ensure that we developed ourselves, our careers, and our strong relationships with our mates before bringing another life into this world. Back then, thirty had seemed so far away. I was secretly sure that one of us would break the rule when we were twenty-eight or so because we both loved babies so much.

By the time my thirtieth birthday rolled around, I was feeling further away from parenthood than ever. And the girlfriend who'd made the promise with me? It was Reyna, who had to skip my party because she couldn't find a sitter and her nannies had quit. She added "mommy" to her list of job titles three whole years ago, while I was still scared to death by even the thought of it.

I bid farewell to my twenties in a blur of mojitos and several karaoked slaughterings of Young MC's "Bust a Move." In my twenties, the clock ticking had been faint, like the stopwatch on *60 Minutes*. Suddenly, it was a gong I could hear over my crappy rap vocal stylings. My fertile years were officially numbered. But it was something else too.

I felt a great sense of nostalgia. For much of my twenties, I was alone. Of course, in retrospect, even the difficult times had taken on a rosy hue. I controlled every aspect of my life. At the time, I bemoaned all the lonely Friday and Saturday nights before I met my husband, spent in my tiny apartment writing, smoking cigarettes, and swilling Diet Coke, listening to Frank Stallone butcher good songs that helped me feel sorry for myself. But part of me loved it. That little apartment was all mine. I answered to no one. I could go to sleep and wake up whenever I wanted to.

Gone were the days of having time to color code my photos then recategorize them by mood. Gone were the hour-long baths reading my favorite sad book, my tears mixing with the bath oils, the soap curling into paisley swirls. Gone were the terrible first dates with the biggest collection of assholes the West Coast had to offer. Men too clichéd to write about—the vain actor, the insecure model, and the broke aspiring musician. And that was just one of them.

Now, I had responsibilities. Now, I did my husband's laundry mixed in with my own. Now, I woke up at six every morning to walk the dog and pick up his poop. Soon, I could be barefoot and pregnant. I would never be alone again. While it was great to be in a wonderful relationship with a man as incredible as my husband, and I loved my dog, I'd never again have the complete freedom that I didn't appreciate in my twenties.

The morning after my big bash, Reyna met me for a walk

to celebrate my birthday belatedly. "So?" Reyna asked me, while pushing baby Sailor in her stroller. "How does it feel to be 30? Embarking on the final frontier of your life?"

"What?" I balked. "Who in the world says 30 is the final frontier?"

"Half of your life is through. The final frontier. The second half."

"Reyna, this isn't the eighteenth century," I said.

Reyna was the worst when it came to parenting public relations. In this way, she was the opposite of Kay. Kay was all about recruitment, Reyna—intentionally or not—always warned about the realities.

She once told me she went an entire week before remembering to brush her teeth, as she had been so busy with her baby when the nannies took their annual week-long vacation.

Today's gem was, "My idea of a romantic date is four hours of uninterrupted sleep."

Every time Reyna said things like this, I secretly wanted to cry. Reyna had wanted to be a mother all her life, just like me. And now she was miserable. "Love my kids, hate motherhood," she always said. Of course, I tried to be a good friend and just listen, but inside, my heart was free-falling like an elevator with its cables cut. Because every

Factoid:

Parenting.com and *Babytalk* magazine polled mothers about what they missed most about their lives prior to having kids. The results showed that 38% said their free time, 27% said their pre-baby bodies, 23% said not having to worry.

time she said that, she hit at the core of my true fear. I was always less concerned about whether I would be a good mom. I always mothered everyone around me—my friends, my dogs, my husband, my brother.

But what if I hated being a mom? Everything else in life was reversible or returnable: jobs, clothing, dogs. But becoming a mom was the one thing you couldn't take back. Knowing that made it almost impossible to take the leap.

In the past, Reyna admitted she and her husband jumped in too soon, getting pregnant on their honeymoon. "You'll be more prepared than I was," she had said.

Then, Reyna stopped in midstride. "Listen to me, Carrie." Her voice was so serious that even little Sailor woke up to hear what her mom had to say. "If anyone tells

---

Factoid:

Parenting.com and *Babytalk* asked women: What is the biggest misconception you had about motherhood before having kids?

- 28% said they thought breastfeeding would come naturally.
- 27% thought their baby weight would come off in a few months.
- 15% thought having a baby would bring the partners closer together.
- 12% thought they could shape their child's personality.
- 10% thought they'd fall in love with their babies at first sight.
- 7% assumed their maternal instincts would kick in right away.

you that all your concerns and worries about parenting just magically disappear when you hold your baby for the first time, you should slap them in the face because they are lying to you. That's a pile of steaming bullshit. Okay?"

I just stared at her in shock. Kay, the parenting public relations goddess, had practically pounded that mantra into my head—that all the fears melted away when you held the baby. Had she been lying? Or was her experience just very different from Reyna's?

"It's bullshit!" Reyna said again for effect, and the tone of her voice startled baby Sailor into a cry. As Reyna continued, I wanted to cry too. "It gets worse!" she said. "You look at this perfect little creature and want to protect her from everything and desperately don't want to screw her up and cause her to go to therapy ever in her life, but you can't. You have the knowledge that the little one will get hurt and knocked around by life, and there's nothing you can do about it. The births of Cayden and Sailor were both the sweetest and most devastating days of my life."

"Well," I said. "Thanks for this pep talk, Rey. I'm just going to drink some Drano and take a nap now."

She hugged me and we laughed, but I knew what she had said was probably true. She walked me back to my house, and I felt as confused as I ever had about becoming a mom. There I was, thirty years old, and it didn't seem to be getting any easier to take the next step. My therapist kept telling me that I would know when I was ready to start a family. Yet I was still lost.

Grampa Carrie

Two days after my birthday, Kay gave birth to her second child. That's right: Maple Leaf became a big brother to—Ariel Drift. It was another boy.

Eight days later, I was holding Ariel at his bris. Because Kay's parents were deceased and Roy's father couldn't make the trip across the country, Kay chose me to be their sandek, which means I got to hold the baby while he got his wee-wee tip snipped—a huge honor.

Have I mentioned I don't do well around blood or any sort of pain? That's a pertinent tidbit to share. Stephen also gets queasy around blood. When we get around to having a child, I imagine we'll both be screaming like teenage girls and shielding our eyes in the delivery room.

I held sweet little eight-day-old Ariel. His tiny fingers curled around my index finger. He slept but moved his mouth a little, like an old man gumming his food. I kissed the top of his head and inhaled that marvelous baby smell, a combination of sweet baby powder and fresh milk. It's mildly addictive. Someone could make a fortune if they bottled this smell—call it "Eau de Bebe"—and sold it in department stores.

You know how they say petting a dog can lower your blood pressure? I've always felt this way about holding babies. I held baby Ariel, rocked him, baby danced with him, and then he opened his eyes. Still adjusting to the light of the world, he looked up at me—and just like that, I was in love with another one of Kay's babies. My tender moment was interrupted by the mohel starting the ceremony.

"And playing the role of Roy's father this morning, Carrie Friedman." The mohel said my last name wrong—emphasized the *Fried* and did so phonetically—which surprised me, since it was a fairly common Jewish last name.

The mohel waited for a laugh that eventually, weakly, came when the few friends gathered realized the mohel was trying to be funny. It was pretty painful stuff, and we hadn't even cut the baby yet.

He then took the baby from me and handed him to Kay, who had to remain seated, as she was still recovering from her emergency c-section. During Kay's water birth, Ariel somehow got caught in her cervix. They made it to the hospital in the nick of time.

The mohel gave me a little wink on his way back to the kitchen counter, his makeshift podium. I swear to you, I had been to almost a dozen brises in the nine years I've lived in Los Angeles and *every single time*, it was the same mohel. He advertised with pamphlets at grocery stores, and I guess it worked. I could've performed his act myself I know his schtick so well. He clearly had unfulfilled entertainment dreams. He spoke to our little group of 10 as if he were addressing a stadium of 3,000.

"May the father rejoice in his offspring, and his mother be glad with the fruit of the loom. I mean her womb." He waited, as if for a rimshot and wild laughter and applause.

While he continued on with his "set," I became transfixed by Kay holding baby Ariel and the way she looked at him. For the first time, I was envious of her—that she had a Maple and an Ariel in her life. I felt a craving to love someone in that way. It wasn't the same as married love. It seemed to be a completely different room in the heart.

A guy I dated once gave me a pillow that had a beautiful Winnie the Pooh quote on it that read, "If you live to be 100, I hope I live to be 100 minus one day, so I never have to live without you." As incredibly sweet as the sentiment was, I was a little creeped out by it, not only because he had given me a Winnie the Pooh pillow when we were both adults, but also because we had only gone on three dates that had proven we lacked even a shred of chemistry. Watching Kay hold her precious son, something snapped into place, and I understood the quote.

Then it was time for the sandek prayer, and Kay handed me the baby. Stephen beamed at me from across the room, and I could tell he liked what he saw. I was flooded with anxiety. I wasn't sure whether it was about parenthood or about the fact that I'd caught a glimpse of the mohel's scalpel on the counter or both. My heart beat faster, my skin got prickly, my forehead beaded with sweat spontaneously. If I weren't thirty, I'd say it was a hot flash. I held onto little Ariel for dear life, all the while telling myself: Don't pass out, don't pass out. Don't drop the baby. That would be a major party foul.

I decided it was a good idea to sit down, but as I sank into the nearest open chair, a few people laughed—better Jews than I was, certainly.

"Look at this! Grampa Carrie just sat on Elijah!" said the mohel, clearly delighted for another moment of comic relief.

Ah yes, the empty chair for the E-man. How could I forget? Sweat dripped down my forehead and into my eyes.

"But seriously, folks," the mohel said, "I was gonna have her sit on Elijah's lap anyway."

Really? "But seriously, folks?" What's next? "I'll be here all week! Try the veal?" The antiperspirant Gods were not smiling on me. Why on this day? Why now? It was just plain cruel, like naming a child Conrad. I was sweating so much my shirt looked like a Rorschach inkblot test. I worried that when I stood up, I'd have what a girlfriend of mine called "Swass," short for ass sweat.

I stood, praying for a dry behind, and handed the baby to the mohel, who announced, "Grampa Carrie will help hold little Ariel while I do my work."

Oh God, I thought. Do I have to? Why can't it be one of the parents? After all, they were the ones who made this baby!

The baby squirmed. The mohel gave me a wine-soaked rag to put in Ariel's mouth to help him with the impending pain.

I tried to focus on the baby, red faced and no bigger than a potato, wiggling and grunting, as if each move, each stretch of his arm, was hard work. He sucked the rag while the mohel made jokes that I tried to tune out. Ariel focused on my face and I smiled at him, trying to keep my eyes up, above his equator, for fear I'd faint if I saw the actual snipping.

Sweet Jesus, I thought ironically. I'm going to pass out.

"And You, God, in Your abounding mercy, send through Your holy angels a holy and pure soul to Ariel Drift, the son of Kay and Roy, who has now been circumcised for the sake of Your great Name. May his heart be open, to learn and to teach, to observe and to practice; grant him long life, a life imbued with the fear of sin, a life of wealth and honor; and fulfill the desires of his heart for good. Amen, and so may it be Your will."

The baby started to cry. And suddenly I was crying too. I wanted to help him. He was looking at me like I had betrayed him. I could have sworn to God he was mouthing the words, "Why didn't you help me, you traitorous bitch!" And I wanted to. More than anything, I wanted to grab this little guy, tuck him close to my chest like a football, and run out of here, past the organic bagels and somehow vegan lox, past the ecologically responsible beet and bean stew, past all the gifts, past the parked cars, and make the pain go away. But I couldn't.

Mercifully the service ended, and I went into the bathroom and wrung out my shirt. Later, I played with Maple, who had gotten cranky because of all the attention his new brother had been getting. I was on the floor of their living room. Maple hid and I pretended I couldn't find him until he popped out from around the corner. "I got you!" he screamed. "You got me!" I screamed back. He laughed and ran, looking back to ensure that I was chasing him. He squealed with delight and kept running—until wham! The worst sight and sound: he tripped over his feet and fell, knocking his face smack on the hardwood floor. As I ran right for him, there was a delay in his response as he took in what had just happened. Then, his face contorted into a full-blown scream and sob.

Of course I gasped, picked him up, held him in my arms, and said, "Oh poor Maple, are you okay?" I hoped to will his pain away.

I had read enough parenting books to know that I had not given the best parental response. If anything, I was supposed to narrate what happened, to allow him to have his own emotions and to feel no need to take on my emotions as well. I remembered when I was a six-year-old tomboy running around and rolling in the grass with friends. At some point I must have cut my knee. As I headed back to our house, my mother saw my bloody knee and screamed, "Oh my GOD, what happened to your leg?" as if it had been shot off. And then what happened? I looked down and unconsciously mirrored my mother's reaction. It *must* be bad, even though it didn't really hurt that much.

Of course, shortly thereafter, Maple dusted himself off and started running again. It took longer for me to recover. I realized this was the root of much of my anxiety: my child would get hurt, both physically and emotionally, and there was nothing I could do about it. I couldn't coat him in rubber or wrap him in rolls of Charmin, as much as I might want to. I couldn't tell off girls who reject him or break his heart.

How could someone bring a child into the world knowing that one day they might—no, will—get hurt or sick? How could I bring a child into this world when I knew I'd eventually have to let him go? Which reminded me of something the author Anne Lamott said, "How on earth can anyone bring a child into this world knowing full well that he or she is eventually going to have to go through the 7th and 8th grades?"

The ages of seven to fifteen were not stellar years for yours truly. Besides having all manner of headgear and comically huge glasses that magnified my eyes and made me look like a hornet, I was just a weird kid in general. In kindergarten and first grade, I was painfully shy and refused to speak. If I wasn't sitting silently in the back of the class, I was drawing elaborate pictures of women in comas. Their faces had stitches and head bandages, with tubes in their noses to help them breathe. My trademark was a single tear streaming down each cheek from their shut eyes. Of course, the teachers called home immediately and asked if there was abuse or if we had any relatives in comas who might be causing me concern. My mother laughed and explained that our cleaning lady had introduced us the summer before to *Days of Our Lives*.

I remember the exact day I lost the unabashed confidence of my youth: I was in the fifth grade, and I liked a boy named Brian who happened to be the most popular boy in school. As a ten-year-old, I still believed every word of parental kindness and support. ("No, those glasses don't look weird! They give your face character!") So, naturally, I assumed I was great. Not better than anyone else, certainly, but I assumed that I was great and that this was universally accepted, even by Brian. Also, I didn't yet understand, nor had I encountered, the heartbreaking situation of liking someone and having those feelings rejected. I would learn this difficult lesson that day.

It was Valentine's Day, and the fifth grade had a tradition in which one could send heart-shaped balloons to their friends or beloved, delivered by an older student dressed as Cupid. I decided this was the perfect event to make my move. This day would be when I'd share my love with Brian and, by association, the world. I bought him three heart-shaped balloons to be delivered individually during last period homeroom. Because he was in a different homeroom than I was, I would not get to witness his no doubt joyous reaction to my declarations of love, but I was sure we could meet up in the hallway when the bell rang at the end of the day.

At the end of last period, I ran down the stairs and into the hallway that held our fifth-grade lockers. I saw Brian at the opposite end of the hall, holding the three balloons, a midair bouquet of what I knew of love at the time. A huge crowd of my fellow students filed out behind him, cheering him on and laughing. I watched as he stuffed the three balloons into his locker and stomped on them ferociously. The pop pop popping of the balloons startled me while everyone laughed. A few people pointed at me. One girl, far more popular than I was, shouted down the hall, "What were you THINKING?"

I had no idea what I'd been thinking. It had never dawned on me that my love wouldn't be returned. It had never dawned on me that everyone had a will of his or her own. I mentally kicked myself for a couple of years after that experience. What *had* I been thinking?

And now I wonder, twenty years later: What will I say to my child when, inevitably, she comes home with her infatuation or love popped as haplessly as those balloons were? What *could* I say? "Yeah, love's incredibly complicated, your heart will no doubt be broken far worse than this someday because 99 out of 100 relationships end"?

My child will fall down and suffer losses and traumas both big and small, and I won't be able to do anything about it. There won't be a way to protect my child from life. That will be the hardest part of parenthood—I already know.

Stephen appeared next to me at the bris reception and said through the side of his mouth, "Don't look now. They've spotted us." I knew exactly whom he was talking about without even looking. We both turned around and smiled to greet Stephen's acquaintance and his wife who, for reference purposes I've dubbed "Mr. and Mrs. Miserable." They were walking reminders of what might happen to us when we had kids.

The husband, Mr. Miserable, said, "Good job, Grampa Carrie! Isn't he a cute baby?"

"Oh, he's adorable!" I said gushing.

Then Mrs. Miserable glared at me and said, "When're you gonna have one?" She sounded annoyed, as though I had offended her in some way by not procreating yet. Everything about this woman was brusque. She grabbed an hors d'oeuvre brusquely, yelled at her hubby brusquely.

"Don't rush them, Doris," the husband said. "God knows, once you've got kids you'll never *not* have them again."

And with that phrase, the avalanche of doom and gloom officially began. Every time we saw them—maybe twice or three times a year—one of them brought up their misery. Usually it was in the form of "Wait 'til you've been married for ten years and have kids." They said it with a tone that implied they thought they were doling out precious words of wisdom, but in truth, they'd become models for us of what not to become.

I'm convinced everyone knows at least one couple like this: the ones who are "staying together because of the kids" and make you want to slit your wrists at the dinner table. They always bicker and snipe in front of us, but about big things, like "Stop draining our bank account!" and "I don't respect you!"

The Miserables' moroseness was amplified, in comparison, by how much Stephen and I were enjoying our time together. We'd just returned from another two-week European vacation, visiting five cities, traipsing and touring, wine tasting and hiking. We'd been working daily to be better partners to each other, develop a strong foundation a language, a shorthand and a division of labor.

Would it all change once we had children? Would we have enough money? Would we ever travel comfortably again? Would we ever have sex again? Or would we become like Mr. and Mrs. Miserable—strangers who happened to live under the same roof and have dinner together?

Was deciding when to add kids to a marriage like locking in at a good interest rate on a house? Sure, you could refinance along the way, with counseling sessions, but wouldn't it be ideal not to have to?

Driving home after the bris, I couldn't get the

Miserables out of my head. Stephen read my expression, turned to me, and said, "It's not foreshadowing, Carrie. Having kids didn't just magically turn them into 'that' couple. We won't turn out like that."

"Can you promise?" I asked.

"Well, no, I guess I can't," he said.

And then I cried.

CHAPTER NINE

Baby Steps ... to Faith

In spite of the six thousand manuals on child raising in the bookstores, child raising is still a dark continent and no one really knows anything. You just need a lot of love and luck—and, of course, courage.

—BILL COSBY

When I came home from a meeting one day, a month after my thirtieth birthday, I couldn't find Bowie the beagle anywhere. Never a good sign. I walked through the house calling his name. By the time I got to the master bedroom, I saw heaps of laundry strewn about. I would have thought I'd been burglarized, but since I couldn't find Bowie anywhere, I knew I'd been Beaglerized.

I followed the trail of clothes, out of which Bowie popped from under a heap. He was camouflaged like E. T. in Drew Barrymore's stuffed animal collection.

The biggest problem with Bowie wasn't his total lack of respect for our authority, rules, or boundaries. No—the

167

biggest problem with Bowie was that he was so physically cute. His little head poking out of the laundry was both aggravating and sweet. He knew what he'd done was wrong because he was shaking like a leaf. He was also playing innocent, which made me want to take a picture of him, not scold him. I continued to follow his trail of destruction into our bathroom, assessing the damage.

The bathroom looked like an old Hollywood crime scene: torn lingerie, an empty pill bottle, the hamper tipped over, as if there had been a struggle. My eyes darted back to the empty pill bottle. I picked it up. Xanax. The same vial of Xanax from my wedding week three years prior. Surely they had lost their efficacy. But then, Bowie heaved and vomited on the bathroom floor.

I blew through stale yellow traffic lights all the way to the vet's office. It had started to drizzle, something so rare in Los Angeles that I would have normally appreciated it, but today it was just another element standing in the way of getting Bowie to the vet. My cell phone rang. My mother.

"Well," she started, "you won't believe who I just saw at the hair salon. Remember your fifth-grade teacher who we always thought was a lesbian?"

"Mom, I can't talk right now, Bowie's sick."

"WHAT?" she shrieked, making the little word a whole three syllables.

"He got into my Xanax," I said. "I'm pulling into the vet right now. Bye." I snapped my phone closed, parked on a diagonal, and ran around and got Bowie out of the back of the car. He lay on his side, looking like a sow about to give birth. He moaned, which could have been from the drugs or the fact that he hated going to the vet.

I ran into the vet's office with Bowie in my arms.

"You again?" the bitch receptionist said.

"Bowie swallowed some pills. I need help."

"Well, how did he get ahold of your pills?" she asked me.

I wanted to slap her. My face was slick with tears and streaks of eye makeup. Couldn't she tell I felt bad enough?

"What did he have and how much?" she asked me. "How many pills were left in the vial?"

"None," I said.

"How many did he eat then?"

Because I took Xanax so infrequently, I had no clue. "It's Xanax that was left over from the weeks leading up to my wedding," I said. "It's three years old. Surely it's expired by now, right?"

"Pills hold their efficacy much longer than their expiration dates indicate."

Well thanks, Negative Nancy. "There were probably 25. Yes, 25 pills." I choked on the words.

And the receptionist had no poker face: "Jesus CHRIST!"

I wanted to tell her I was so sick of her condescending comments and judgments over these last few years. I wanted to tell her she was a horrid person and shouldn't work at a vet, where kindness was required as most people loved their pets like family. I wanted to tell her that after today, no matter what happened, I'd never come back to this place. I'd drive twenty minutes to another vet if I had to, just so I could avoid her shitty attitude.

But I didn't say any of those things. I just yelled, "GET ME A DOCTOR, NOW."

She made us wait. I held Bowie like a baby, all forty pounds of him spilling over my lap. I thought after ingesting Xanax, he'd be calm. He was the opposite—panting and trembling. I tried to calm myself down so that he couldn't feel my anxiety and tension. I gently rocked him. He looked up at me and licked my face. He had placed his trust in me, and I had failed him. His licking felt like a final plea, "Please, I promise I won't be bad, Mom." I couldn't hold him tight enough.

But then a nurse came to take him away.

"We need to pump his stomach," she said.

She took his leash and pulled him away from me. Bowie put on his brakes as they dragged him through two steel doors. He looked back at me the whole way. I nodded at him feebly, as if that might reassure him that I approved of these people who were taking him away. He always did this, every time I left him anywhere. In those dark beginning days with Bowie, I had entertained the possibility of giving him away to someone with a larger yard or higher level of patience. But I knew I would never forget the image of him looking back at me, searching for my love and reassurance. I thought that I could eventually get over my love for Bowie if I needed to. But watching them take Bowie away, I knew I could never do it.

I understood why I had been so scared of loving something this much. In times of panic, unconditional love seems like a bad investment, but with Bowie, there was no other choice. Bowie always managed to wriggle under the covers, ending up between us, with his head on our pillows, snoring away. He opened another door—hell, a whole new wing—in my heart.

I sat in the waiting room, watching people come and go. Some cried as they left with empty animal carriers. I prayed that wouldn't be my fate.

I tried to flip through the clinic's wide array of *Cat Fancy* magazines from 2002, but I was preoccupied by my sad, guilty, terrified thoughts. How could I be a mother if I couldn't even handle this dog? I had voiced this concern before, but friends of mine, over the years, had refuted it,

"When I picked up Millie at the animal shelter, she was sick and suffering. That first afternoon home, she put her head on my lap and fell asleep. The trust she placed in me to protect her and care for her when she could not care for herself was overwhelming, overpowering. I thought to myself that I could never love another being more. Now, she sleeps with me every night. She wakes me up in the morning to let me know she needs to go outside by licking my hand or cheek. She's insistent but gentle. Usually, in those first few minutes between sleeping and waking, I nuzzle her neck or her belly. In those moments, it is like we share a soul."

—V.K., Albuquerque, NM

saying that Bowie was the equivalent of an eighteen-month-old baby permanently arrested at that stage of development. Even dog trainers we had worked with had suggested that Bowie was more challenging than most dogs. He had eaten up a lot of our money. Literally—he had eaten cash. He once ran into my den, tail wagging gleefully, with half a $20 bill in his mouth. In the span of less than two minutes, he had pulled my purse off the kitchen counter and, like a teenager, raided it for money and gum. But none of this made me feel any better.

My phone rang again. This time, it was my brother.

"Billy," I said, "I can't talk right now—"

"Carrie! You had Xanax and didn't share it with me? What kind of sister are you?" he teased. Then he hung up on me. This was how fast news traveled through our family network. Mom called my brother, he sent a text to his girlfriend, my father, sister, and her husband. And now, the enmeshment circus had come to town: my phone was lighting up with messages and texts from all of them. "We R Praying 4 BoBo" and "U need 2 B more careful w/ ur meds."

Finally, after an hour that felt like seven, the doctor came out and motioned for me to follow him. I tried to swallow the lump in my throat. He took me into a small and empty sterile room. "Where's Bowie?" I asked, my voice cracking.

The doctor said, "He ingested a lot of drugs." He spoke far more gently than he'd ever spoken to me before, and I knew it was bad news. The tears came, and they didn't stop.

The vet spoke but I didn't hear him; I just watched his scary red unibrow lift and lower like the arm at a tollbooth. Stephen called him "Beaker" at home, because of his general muppetiness.

"I need to see him," I said, interrupting the doctor. "I need to see him now."

"Okay," he said. "He's in here." He led me past the nurse's station and into another small, cold room. "I'll give you a moment with him." A moment: so fleeting, so finite. I wiped my cheeks with the backs of my hands.

There, on the table, was my Bowie, my little boy, lying on his side. He had an IV in his front leg and stickers that looked like little round Band-Aids with wires that attached to a machine tracking his heartbeat. I pulled a chair next to the table and petted him where I thought I wouldn't hurt him or interfere with any of his tubes and wires. I rubbed parts of his belly, the palomino patch of pink and brown freckles. He always loved his belly rubs. He looked at me. His blinks were too long for my taste; his girlish long eyelashes batting slowly. I was mentally taking back every bad thing I had ever said or thought about him, as if this would help my cause in some way. I used to joke that I liked Bowie best when he was sleeping. Now, all I wanted was for him to wake up.

I could tell he was fading. I did not want to yell for the doctor, because if these were my Bowie's last moments, I wanted him to feel safe and peaceful. I cradled his head, watching the longer breaks between each of his blinks. Despite my initial reluctance to let this dog into my heart, he had become such a mama's boy. He had never wavered in his love for me. He had given it unconditionally since the day I met him over two years before. Perhaps he could sense that I was a challenge and I was holding out. Or maybe it was because I was the one who opened his cans of dog food.

I got very close to his ear and talked to him in order to keep him awake. I said anything. I said everything. "I love you so much, Bowie peanuts. Your daddy loves you so much. You're such a good boy. You're your mom's best boy."

And then he closed his eyes. I cried so hard it hurt. I cried so hard I couldn't hold my head up. This was my fault, my mistake. I was an awful mother.

Then, something came over me. I stopped crying and instantly turned into Shirley MacLaine in *Terms of Endearment*.

I ran out of the little room and yelled, "Help! Help! He's crashing! Save him! You have to save him! PLEASE!" I banged on the desk at the nurses' station. "He's dying! My dog—please, wake him up! Resuscitate him!"

The doctor and a nurse came over, both looking alarmed and confused.

"He's not dying," Beaker said.

"Huh?" I asked.

"He's not dying. He's falling asleep. He still has a little bit of Xanax in his system. But he will be fine now. We pumped his stomach, and he is just sleeping off the little bit left in his bloodstream."

"Well. Someone should have mentioned that when I came in." It was tempting to add "douche bag" to the end of that sentence, but I was too relieved that sweet Bo would live. I slid down the wall and heaved a sigh of relief.

The Dark

I've learned three undeniable truths during my years on this earth:

1. Most independent films are depressing.
2. Anyone who calls their job a "gig" can't pay for dinner.
3. Human beings fear the unknown.

I was terrified of the dark as a kid, certain that some horrible monster would pop out of the great, threatening abyss. I still am. When I enter a room, I hold my breath until I've turned on a light and burrow under the bed covers once they're out at nighttime.

I've always felt lost and desperate when I'm not in control. I was the kid who bit the puzzle pieces to make them fit. I've gathered that parenthood is most definitely a journey into the unknown.

A girlfriend of mine from college called. We hadn't connected in far too long. She had two little boys now—one was three, one was eighteen months. Both, I learned in this phone call, were profoundly autistic. She didn't say this breezily and certainly didn't take it lightly, but she also seemed to have come to terms with it.

I didn't know what to say when she told me. "I'm sorry" didn't feel right, especially since she didn't sound upset. So I asked her to tell me about them, and she did. They're hitting all their milestones much later than normal, but it didn't make it any less incredible when they did. She had no help except for the behavioral therapists she took her boys to twice a week.

The most amazing part of the story: she was pregnant again. She had two children who required all her time and attention, and she was tickled pink to be having another.

"Having a child is an opportunity," she said. "An opportunity to affect the world. I will be contributing three well-raised members to society. And I've been given the opportunity to help my boys. These were the kids I was meant to have and raise. I love them. They are who they are."

"How do you do it?" I asked her. What I didn't ask her was, how did she have the courage and the conviction to try again?

"You rise to the occasion," she said. "You have no idea what you're capable of until you're challenged. You'll surprise yourself. Nothing ever goes the way you plan it, so let go of that idea right now."

I thought about all the expectations and hopes we naturally placed on our unborn kids.

"Like George Michael says, you've got to have faith," she said with a laugh.

Faith in what, I wondered to myself. Usually, I don't "do" faith. Don't get me wrong—my life is full of gifts: my husband is truly the soul mate I was meant to find; we have shelter, we have jobs we love, and we don't go to bed hungry. These aren't small things, especially in today's world. Part of me wonders, in all our happiness, if maybe we should quit while we're ahead.

But after talking to this friend of mine, I was in awe: she did everything right and had gotten this result twice, yet she still had faith in the world and herself. It made me wonder how she, and so many other people, continued to take this leap anyway, knowing that something so unexpected could occur. How do we relinquish control and learn to trust ourselves, our relationships, and our instincts? How do we accept the natural order of things?

As soon as I asked myself these questions, my perspective shifted. I didn't even have any answers, but I could breathe a little easier, the tightness in my chest had disappeared. All the kids I saw on the street and in cafés were well-behaved and their parents looked relatively happy too.

The shift sneaked up on me in surprising moments. I was at the grocery store in the vitamin aisle. I loved this particular store because they often had two-for-one deals on vitamins.

I saw a little boy who couldn't have been more than three years old walking with his mom. His hair was going every which way, and he had clearly dressed himself, wearing purple and four different shades of blue. Three primary-colored balloons were tied to his wrist. And his mom walked slightly in front of him, asking him what colors they were and what shape a balloon was.

The boy with the balloons, trailing slightly behind her, yelled "MOMMY! I think I'm gonna fly away! Whoooa!"

His mother turned around and laughed, took him by the hand, and said, "Well, take me with you! I wanna come with you!"

I watched this from the vitamin aisle, then burst into tears. The boy with the balloons walked off with his mother, leaving me wiping my face. I scanned the rows of pills. I was searching for something but wasn't entirely sure that I knew what. It was as if my heart was in on the secret, but my brain wasn't. Without thinking, I placed two bottles of prenatal vitamins into my shopping cart. The expiration dates were in a year and a half. Surely I'd be ready to use them before then. My action made no sense. But for once, I wasn't thinking. I was feeling.

Training Wheels

My father often reminds me of the day I learned to ride a bicycle. I don't need to be reminded. I remember it well.

I came late to the world of bike riding. My friends were riding around long before I was. I had tried it without the training wheels a few times before, but I hated the unpredictability, the precariousness. Like the balance beams in gym class, I didn't quite understand the point. Why make walking or getting somewhere more difficult by doing it on a thin elevated bar or on two slim rubber wheels?

One day, at the age of seven years old, I decided it was time to bite the bullet. I was tired of not being able to join

---

"The hardest part of raising a child is teaching them to ride bicycles. A shaky child on a bicycle for the first time needs both support and freedom. The realization that this is what the child will always need can hit hard."

—Sloan Wilson

the local kids at the nearby park for their version of off-roading. I had to learn. I wanted to learn.

That day, with my father behind me, holding lightly onto the back of the bike seat, I kept falling off, skinning my knees, and tearing holes into my pants. It went like this for hours, but I refused to give up. At one point, my dad went inside to take a business call. As I waited on the bike, I looked down at the pedals. I put one foot and then the other on them. Then I pushed them down one at a time. Suddenly, I was doing it—I had conquered it. I was riding a bike all by myself! I still remember the pride I felt pulsing in my chest. I was literally going places! When my father came back outside, I was an official bike rider. I'll never forget the proud look on my dad's face.

I was soaring up and down our driveway. The wind running through my hair; I even got fancy and lifted one hand off the handlebars to wave to our neighbor. Then I rang the bell. Of course, I finally stopped when I crashed into a brick wall. I nearly broke my face because I hadn't learned how to use the brakes yet. Even though bike riding was terrifying and painful, I loved every minute of it and got right back on the bike to do it again.

I was eating lunch at a Mexican chain restaurant and

> "I was awake for the whole thing and it took her awhile to breathe once she was taken out . . . which was like, the worst moment of my life. But once I heard that little cry, both of us were a mess of tears. Then they showed her to me and, man, people aren't kidding. . . . She was the most beautiful creature I had ever seen."
>
> —G.K., Westchester, CA

trying not to watch a man two booths away inhaling a cup of salsa with a spoon, scooping it into his mouth in wince-worthy helpings.

A mother came in with a tiny baby in a front pack and sat in an adjacent booth. From her tired eyes and her weary waddle, I guessed she wasn't necessarily a lady who lunches but, rather, a very new mom. She noticed Salsa Man and then averted her gaze and busied herself with her baby. She unfolded a travel bassinet and placed the baby in it. The baby carried on and screamed.

Salsa Man stared at the mother, who lifted her baby back up in a protective gesture, which left her without a free hand to eat with. She put her head down and tried to pick up individual pieces of lettuce with her mouth, as if bobbing for apples.

Normally, I would have felt a mixture of annoyance and anxiety, but I'd been feeling differently lately. Instead of ignoring the new mother and her baby, I wanted to help them. I got up from my booth, walked past skeevy Salsa Man, and asked the mom if she needed someone to spell her for a second.

"Oh, thank you," she said. "Please. I just, I'm going to faint if I don't eat something soon."

"No problem. I'll stand right here and hold her." The mother handed her baby over to me and gratefully ate her lunch.

The baby looked at me as if deciding whether to cry. I rubbed her back. "Oh, sweet one," I said. "It's okay." I willed her not to cry, not to reinforce my fears of my inability to parent.

"Grace," her mother told me when I asked. "Her name is Grace."

Grace, this little peanut of a babe, rested her head

against my shoulder. I baby danced with her for ten minutes, cooing and singing the little songs I made up as I went along. Suddenly, I was a little girl playing with my dolls and then a teenager babysitting those five wonderful boys.

The questions about becoming a mother, for me, had never been IF, but, rather, when, why, and how. But standing in that noisy chain restaurant, all my questions momentarily flew out the window, and it was just me and baby Grace looking in each other's eyes.

I still had more questions than answers. But I'd finally accepted that some questions can't ever be answered. Having children is the biggest leap a person can take. All this time, I had thought I wasn't ready. But maybe no one's ever quite ready. There was never going to be a perfect time to start a family, but everything worth having and doing required risk and courage.

Later that night, while Stephen and Bowie slept in our bed, I took my first prenatal vitamin.

Acknowledgments

This book would not have been possible if Newsweek hadn't published my essay in the summer of 2007. I thank them and everyone who responded to my article for inspiring me to write this book.

I interviewed a vast number of incredible women and men for this book and am extremely grateful for their time, generosity, and thoughts. I thank my agent, Stacey Glick, for her tireless efforts and persistence. I don't have the words to express how much I want to thank my editor, Danielle Chiotti (though, being the brilliant editor she is, she'd probably find those perfect words). I also want to thank Amy Pyle and everyone at Kensington for acting as the glue that holds this book together more firmly than the binding.

Many thanks to my earliest readers for being brutally honest, and to my friends and sister, Meggan, my mother, Lili, and my brother, Andrew, for indulging in lengthy discussions with me and offering terrific insights. And I can't forget the great Nicky Weinstock, who introduced me to Jane and Miriam in the first place.

A final thank you to my phenomenal husband for buoying me with his love, patience, and support all these years.